ORGANIC BODY CARE RECIPES

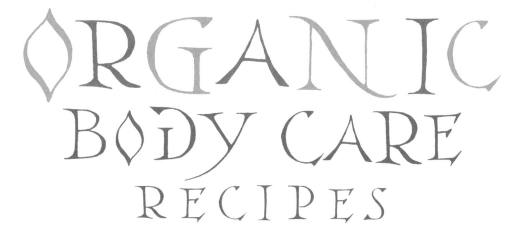

175 Homemade Herbal Formulas for Glowing Skin & a Vibrant Self

Stephanie Tourles

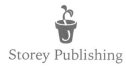

Storey Publishing

The mission of Storey Publishing is to serve our customers by publishing practical information that encourages personal independence in harmony with the environment.

Edited by Deborah Balmuth and Elaine M. Cissi
Art direction and text design by Mary Winkelman Velgos
Cover and concept design by Stewart A. Williams
Text production by Liseann Karandisecky
Illustrations by Kathy Bray: 11; Alison Kolesar: 7, 14, 209; and Laura Tedeschi:
36, 46, 47, 60, 63, 65, 67, 71, 72, 75, 77, 78, 81, 83, 85, 86, 89, 90, 92, 125, 172
Author photo by Janice Semprini
Indexed by Index Arts

Printed in the United States by R.R. Donnelley
10 9 8 7 6 5 4 3 2 1

Library of Congress Cataloging-in-Publication Data

Tourles, Stephanie L., 1962–
    Organic body care recipes / by Stephanie Tourles.
        p. cm.
    Rev. ed of: The herbal body book. c1994.
    ISBN 978-1-58017-676-7 (pbk. : alk. paper)
    1. Beauty, Personal. 2. Herbal cosmetics.
    I. Tourles, Stephanie L., 1962– Herbal body book. II. Title.
RA778.T64 2007
613'.488—dc22
                                                                    2007009814

To my Willy

Here's to the second half of our lives.
May our love blossom and flourish, being as
sweet and succulent as a handful of fresh-picked,
shiny black huckleberries in August.

Contents

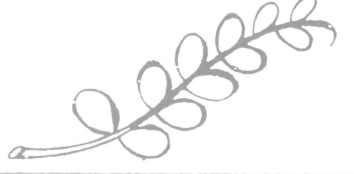

Acknowledgments

To all the gardeners; herbalists; aromatherapists; biologists; landscapers; farmers; cosmetic chemists; elders of the past; and even the plants themselves, my lifelong teachers of the green world who have shared their wisdom with me over the years: Without you, this book would have been impossible and my green soul would not be fulfilled.

I am also eternally grateful to those of you who have been my cosmetic "guinea pigs" over the years — friends, family members, and complete strangers who have allowed me to apply my new personal care concoctions to your faces, arms, legs, hands, feet, backs, and hair, and who have given me in return valued feedback toward the perfection of my formulations. "Practice makes perfect," so the saying goes . . . and some of you knew when to tell me that an experimental cream, mask, or massage oil was either far from perfect or that it was positively perfect and produced the desired result. I made meticulous notes of your observations, good and bad.

Speaking of far from perfect, I remember the dreaded blueberry-mask experiment of my early years: This sweetly fragranced fruit mask, high in beneficial antioxidants and supposedly pampering to the skin, turned a work associate's skin supremely soft — and also, regretfully, a lovely shade of pale blue! At least she had a sense of humor — thank goodness! Live, learn, and laugh, I say! Without everyone's comments and patience I could not have gained the knowledge necessary to become the natural cosmetic chemist and holistic esthetician that I am today. I thank you all.

Introduction

Did you know that women use an average of 12 personal care products daily? And men aren't far behind, with about seven in their daily routine. Each day we use soap, body scrub, lotion, face cleanser, toner, night cream, shave cream, after-shave balm, sunscreen, makeup, and deodorant, so it's important to know what's coming into contact with our skin. Remember: Your skin eats — or, more accurately, absorbs.

The official term for the process of absorption of substances via the skin is *transdermic penetration.* All topical substances can either penetrate or affect the skin's surface. To what degree depends on the particular substance, molecular size of the ingredient(s), temperature, and the condition of the skin at the time of contact.

If you're having a hard time believing that your skin can actually absorb some of the ingredients from your favorite body product, then you have only to think of three popular drugs that are transported into the bloodstream via a topically applied patch: nicotine used for cessation of smoking, hormones for birth control, and nitroglycerin for angina pectoris.

As a licensed esthetician and holistic skin care specialist, my focus is on educating individuals so that they can realize their highest health and beauty potential through the use of natural skin and body care products and vitalizing lifestyle habits. I want my clients and readers to become active participants in their own well-being.

In my years of experience, I have worked with a wide range of commercially prepared products, including high-end preparations and "natural" products from health food stores and wellness spas. Many of these skin and body care preparations, even the so-called natural ones, contain highly toxic and irritating ingredients. Frequently, I've heard from both clients and my readers who have endured allergic reactions or other skin sensitivities resulting from their use of these often costly and often synthetic products.

But if potentially irritating or harmful chemicals and artificial colorants and fragrances can be absorbed by your skin, then so can highly beneficial natural ingredients, which can promote beauty and wellness.

In this rapidly advancing technological age of skin and body care, you can visit your local medical spa and choose from a dizzying array of "youthifiers." A few of the products and services offered might be pharmaceutically enhanced cosmetics; laser skin resurfacing; acid-based skin peels; microdermabrasion; surgical face and body reconstruction; permanent hair removal; application of permanent eye and lip liner and brow color; intense pulsed light for acne treatment; or an injection cocktail to temporarily remove this, that, or the other wrinkle.

While these technological advancements do have their place, they shouldn't prevent us from taking control of our own bodies. These quick fixes do not come without some pain, risk, or high cost. Nor do they offer an everlasting cure-all to our perceived physical or emotional shortcomings.

The time is ripe for getting back to the basics. Many of us have lost sight of our true selves in an effort to become synthesized, smoothed, or physically augmented. It's important to remember, however, that Hollywood hype is *not* reality — nor should it be.

Holistic herbal skin and body care comprises an ancient tradition practiced for thousands of years, promoting mutual respect between individuals and generations; harmony and balance within; gentle coexistence with the earth; and a visible physical radiance in the individuals who practice it. Herbs and other

THE HIGH PRICE OF VANITY

According to Myra Michelle Eby, founder of MyChelle Dermaceuticals, a large number of the chemicals and artificial fragrances in our daily applications of body care products have names that might sound like Greek to us — but because our skin may absorb up to 60 percent of them, they can all be potentially harmful. Once in our bodies, our fatty tissue stores these chemicals, leading to a host of possible problems. The solution to avoiding these chemicals: Read the label!

Parabens, "estrogen mimickers and chemical preservatives found in almost all body care products," as Eby puts it, can affect those who have what's known as paraben-mix allergy, resulting in rashes after applying a product. In fact, some topical parabens have even been detected in human breast tumors! In addition, paraben allergic sensitivity is not uncommon.

Other preservatives such *as DMDM hydantoin, imidazolidinyl urea and quaternium 15* are very common and can release trace amounts of formaldehyde into the skin, leading to joint discomfort and contact dermatitis.

The chemical *triethanolamine (TEA),* often used as a base for cleansers and in cosmetics to adjust pH, may cause allergic reactions, skin and hair dryness, and eye irritations.

Artificial fragrances are often manufactured from petrochemicals and can irritate the skin and strip it of its natural protection and even lead to difficulties such as headaches and asthmatic complications.

Synthetic colors such as FD&C or D&C followed by a number can be carcinogenic. Fortunately, some commercial products do have natural coloring agents.

Phthalates, which can accumulate in the skin and lead to an increased risk of reproductive abnormalities, can be found in hair sprays, perfumes, and nail polish.

natural ingredients are nourishing, pampering, cleansing, protective, and fragrant to body and soul. They produce in us a profound sense of authentic beauty, contentment, and well-being.

With the instructions and recipes in this book, you'll learn how to create natural, often organic personal care products for skin, hair, and nails that sing with vitality, vibrance, and inner wellness. The formulas I've created will help correct current skin problems and prevent future ones, smooth and balance your skin, pamper and fragrance your body, entice your significant other, and address some intimate-care issues. Natural, simple, cost-effective remedies can be the basis for long-term skin and body care!

As you'll learn, the consistent practice of holistic health, beauty, and lifestyle habits is always the key to looking and feeling your best. But don't forget to have some fun along the way, too. Whether you're new to making handmade personal care products or are highly skilled at cosmetic cookery, keep in mind that these recipes are designed to be relatively easy to make, pleasurable to use, and simple to customize according to your needs or whim. Many make great gifts, too.

May your journey with herbs and other pure, natural ingredients bring you endless joy and delight and the realization that your body is a beautiful and faithful friend to your spirit.

DID YOU KNOW?

The molecular structure of a pure plant essential oil — one of the many plant derivatives with skin healing properties used in the formulas in this book — is so small that within minutes after application, the oil can be detected on the breath and in the bloodstream! Just imagine what benefits your skin will receive from the rapid absorption of these regenerative and beautifying wonders of nature!

ONE

A Natural Approach to Beautiful Skin, Hair, and Nails

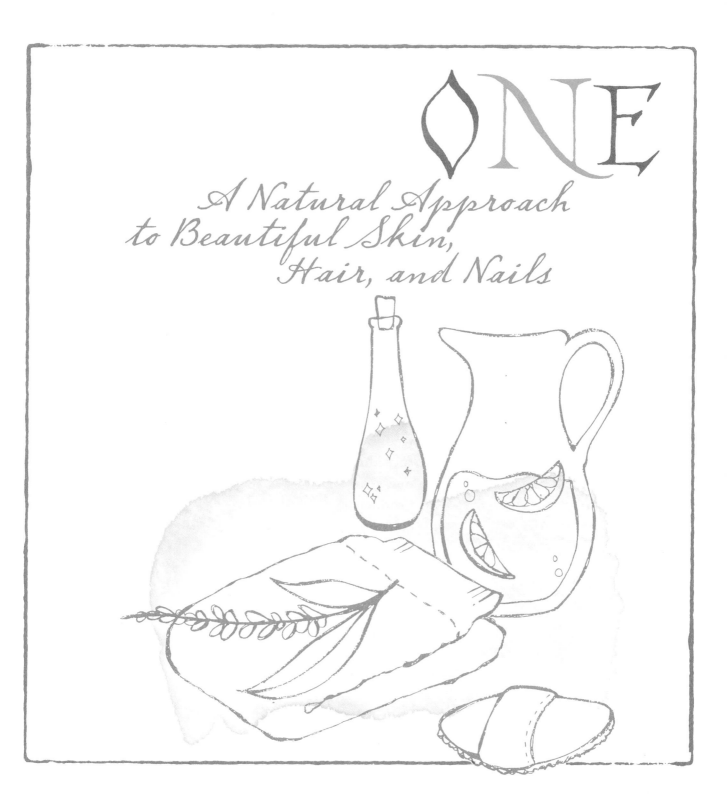

In order to care properly for your skin, hair, and nails, it's important that you understand something about their structure and purpose. Knowing how, why, and when to care for them and identifying the best formulas for their needs will help them remain healthy and beautiful regardless of the climate you live in or your chronological age.

Your Skin

Think of your skin as a beautiful, satin robe that you wear night and day. It presents your external beauty and health to the world and at the same time protects your inner being. The skin, or integumentary system, is an actual *living system* that also comprises the hair and nails, various glands, and several specialized receptors. As a complex structure, it performs nine essential jobs for the body. The skin:

- Protects us from physical, chemical, biological, thermal, and electrical damage.
- Helps the body maintain a steady temperature.
- Acts as a moisture regulator, preventing excessive entry and evaporation of water.
- Prevents excessive loss of minerals.
- Converts ultraviolet rays into vitamin D3, part of the vitamin D complex that helps us maintain strong bones by enhancing absorption of calcium and other minerals.
- Serves as a highly sensitive sensory organ, responding to heat, cold, pain, pleasure, and pressure.
- Metabolizes and stores fat.
- Secretes sebum, an oily lubricating substance.
- Assists in processes of excretion of salts, urea, water, and toxins via sweating.

As a general rule, your skin is designed to keep out more things than it lets in, though openings in the surface from burns, abrasions, cuts, pimples, ulcers, boils, or acne can allow infectious bacteria to enter. Its follicular openings and pores also allow some topically applied substances to be absorbed.

Helpful to us, our skin constantly transmits and receives information. If something is amiss, it displays signs of interior or exterior distress. If all is well, it displays radiance.

The *cutis,* or skin, is our largest body organ; it consists of tissues structurally joined together to perform specific activities. The thickness of this organ varies: The skin on the eyelids and scrotum are the thinnest — thinner even than the paper these words are printed on — and the skin on the soles of your feet and your palms is the thickest. The skin of an average-sized adult weighs approximately five to eight pounds and, if stretched out flat, would cover an area approximately 17 to 20 square feet.

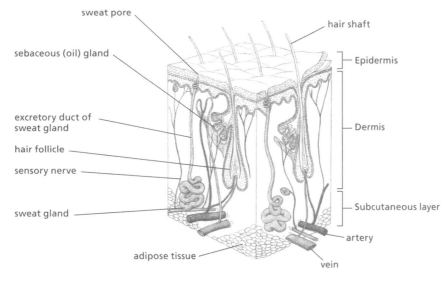

sweat pore
hair shaft
sebaceous (oil) gland
Epidermis
excretory duct of sweat gland
Dermis
hair follicle
sensory nerve
sweat gland
Subcutaneous layer
adipose tissue
artery
vein

A cross section of skin

Of the three layers of skin — epidermal, dermal, and subcutaneous — the epidermal layer, or *epidermis* (also known as the *cuticle* or *scarf skin*) is the outermost, thinnest layer. Though it contains no blood vessels, it does have many small nerve endings and shows the world your wrinkles, break-outs, dry flakes, laugh lines, sunburns, blisters, age spots, and freckles — in other words, the results of genetics and lifestyle habits, good and bad.

The epidermis consists of a soft form of *keratin proteins* (hair, fingernails, and toenails are made of hard keratin) which are resistant to water and many chemicals and provide a shield of protection from the outside world. The *melanocytes*, or cells that produce your skin's particular pigment, are also found in the epidermis.

The dermal layer, or *dermis* (also known as the *corium* or *true skin*) lies just below the epidermis and is a tough elastic layer of connective tissue. Its abundant blood supply puts roses in your cheeks and gives you a look of vitality. This strong, yet flexible, layer holds together your internal organs, bones, fluids, and so forth.

The two major components of the dermis are *collagen* and *elastin* — fibers that impart the skin's strength and resilience. According to some studies, wrinkles begin in the dermis due to a

Testing Your Age

Want to know your skin's biological age? In her book *Natural Hand Care* (Storey Publishing, 1998), Norma Pasekoff Weinberg offers this experiment to test the elasticity or stretchability of your skin.

Pinch the skin on the back of your hand, and then release it after a few seconds. If you're under 30 years of age, the skin will quickly return to its original contour. If you are between 30 and 50, you can begin to see the skin stand up for a second or two before recovering. At age 50 and beyond, the skin may stand up for a number of seconds, a sign that its support network has been altered or that the body as a whole is undergoing changes that are visible at the skin's surface.

change in elastin causing its structure to lose its snap. The result is that skin becomes slack, like an old rubber band. Some skin professionals believe that wrinkles are due to a degeneration of collagen, the protein providing the skin's strength and form. Maybe someday science will discover the true physiological process that leads to wrinkling, but for now, we know only that without sufficient moisture, the collagen and elastin matrix loses its ability to keep skin toned and supple.

As we age, skin naturally thins, its elastin weakens, and collagen production slows. Abuse of skin care products or neglect of basic care; poor nutrition; lack of hydration; insufficient exercise; and excessive exposure to sun, salt, wind, pollution, and dry air can also take their toll. Emotional stressors such as anger, depression, deep sadness, relationship issues, and the death of loved ones add to the chemical changes that occur within your body and appear on your skin.

The third layer of skin, the subcutaneous layer, or *subcutis,* is the fatty or *adipose* layer that lies beneath the dermis and connects to the underlying muscle tissue. A little fat is a good thing as far as your skin is concerned. It keeps your face from looking drawn and hollow and gives your body beautiful contours

WHAT'S CONTAINED IN ONE SQUARE INCH OF SKIN

The complex structures of the skin contained within one square inch:

- 65 hairs
- 9,500,000 cells
- 95 to 100 sebaceous (oil) glands
- 19 yards (17 meters) of blood vessels
- 650 sweat glands
- 78 yards (70 meters) of nerves
- 78 sensory apparatuses for heat
- 19,500 sensory cells at the ends of nerve fibers
- 1,300 nerve endings to record pain
- 160 to 165 pressure apparatuses for the perception of tactile stimuli
- 13 sensory apparatuses for cold

Adapted from Joel Gerson, *Milady's Standard Textbook for Professional Estheticians*, eighth edition.

and smoothness. Fat provides a strong foundation for your skin and acts as a shock absorber and insulator protecting your internal organs. Circulation is maintained here by a network of arteries and lymphatics. This adipose layer provides your entire body with a storage house of vital, long-term energy reserves to draw upon as necessary. As you age (or crash diet), the subcutis becomes thinner, leaving behind sagging, unsupported skin.

Your Hair

Hair, or *pilus*, is an appendage of the skin — slender, threadlike outgrowths of fiber that extend through follicular openings within the skin and scalp. Hair grows over the entire body, with the exception of the soles of your feet, palms of your hands, lips, and eyelids. It is made of approximately 97 percent protein (keratin) and 3 percent moisture.

When treating the hair's internal and external structure, keep in mind these two substances: protein (to fortify, strengthen, and encourage growth) and water or moisture (to hydrate). The hair shaft, that part that extends from the scalp, has become *keratinized*, or hardened. It has no nerves, blood, or muscles. While the hair on your head provides some insulation from heat, cold, and sun, its main purpose may be purely ornamental.

The hair shaft has three distinct layers: the *cuticle, cortex,* and *medulla.* The *cuticle,* or outermost layer, is the part you see. It's your hair's coat of armor and is composed of overlapping scales that appear much like the shingles on a roof. When these lie flat, they reflect light and your hair appears shiny. When the cuticle is roughened due to damage resulting from hot styling implements, chemical treatments, medications, poor-quality styling aids, excessive teasing and brushing, and environmental stress, it appears dull and perhaps flyaway and frizzy.

The *cortex*, or middle layer of hair, is constructed of elongated cells or parallel fibers of hard proteins that grow end on end instead of scalelike. These cells give hair its flexibility and tensile strength. Due to protein and water content, the cortex comprises approximately 90 percent of the hair's molecular weight. Here you'll find the pigments, or *melanin*, that determine your natural color. Hair turns gray because the source of melanin has been depleted.

The parallel protein fibers in the cortex are held together by a variety of bonds. The greatest number are hydrogen bonds, which can be mechanically broken by the use of brushes, combs, rollers, curling irons, and flat irons. The strongest of the bonds, disulfide bonds, can be broken only by chemical means such as those used in straightening, perming, highlighting, or coloring. Your crowning glory can become structurally weak when large numbers of bonds are broken and not are reformed. This can lead to permanent damage that must be at least regularly trimmed.

The *medulla,* or innermost layer of a hair, is composed of protein. Its health contributes to hair's body and elasticity and it may be entirely absent in very fine hair.

We can keep all of this information in mind the next time we submit our hair to torture in the name of vanity. A simple, uncompromising beauty routine is important to both our hair's health and our good looks.

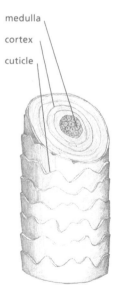

medulla
cortex
cuticle

**A cross section
of the hair strand**

A Healthy Root = Healthy Hair

Every hair on your body grows from a living root, or *papilla*, embedded in the dermis at the base of the hair follicle. This is where the newly forming hair makes a connection with the rest of the body via the bloodstream. Good circulation in the scalp is essential to a healthy head of hair; it allows an ample supply of oxygenated, nutrient-rich blood to reach the root and encourage growth. The scalp, like your toes and fingers, is one of the hardest places on your body for blood to reach. A daily scalp massage is not merely an indulgence, but an important beauty ritual!

If you're in good health, your hair will grow with glossy ease. But toxins, drugs, poor diet, lack of exercise, hormonal fluctuations, and ill health are also reflected at the hair's root. The volume, body, shine, rate of growth, and general health of your hair and scalp are dependent on the food and water received by the hair's root. One of the primary reasons for hair loss and premature graying is a lack of nourishment. Proper diet, regular scalp stimulation, and removal of follicle-clogging sebum are the three keys to a glorious crop of hair.

HAIR FACTS

Lorraine Massey and Deborah Chiel, authors of the book *Curly Girl* (Workman, 2001), explain that hair grows at a rate of about one half inch a month. A follicle will keep growing a hair for three to five years. When it stops, the follicle enters a period of rest for a few weeks while the hair root is released. Right after this, the hair falls out. Every day we lose about one hundred hairs of the roughly one hundred thousand we have on our head at any given time. Just days after one hair falls out, the follicle begins growing a replacement.

Your Nails

Like hair, fingernails and toenails are appendages of the skin. The nail, or *onyx*, composed of the hardest keratin, exists to protect the ends of the fingers and toes, help your fingers grasp small objects, aid in general grooming, and scratch an itch. The average growth rate of an adult fingernail is approximately one-eighth inch per month; toenails grow more slowly.

The *nail body*, or *plate*, is the visible surface of the nail that's attached to the skin beneath it. The *free edge* is the portion of the nail that extends beyond the tip of the finger or toe — the part that you cut or file. Though it appears as a single structure, the nail is actually made up of many layers.

The *nail bed*, lying beneath the surface of the nail body, is richly supplied with blood vessels (it should appear pink in color) which provide nourishment necessary for nail growth. There is also a wealth of nerve endings in this area.

The *nail root* is embedded at the base of the nail, just above the *nail matrix*. This is where nail growth begins, with the rate determined by the nutrients it receives. Matrix cells produce the keratin that becomes the visible nail. This highly sensitive area also contains nerves, blood vessels, and lymph vessels. If the matrix is irreparably injured, irregular nail growth results.

The *lunula* is the pale "half moon" at the base of the nail that serves as a semi-transparent window through which to see the nail root and matrix beneath. This crescent is nearly always visible on the thumbs, but may be less or not at all visible on the other fingers.

The *cuticle* is the small flap of skin that often hangs over the nail plate, protecting the delicate matrix below. It's important to remember *never* to cut your cuticles or let a nail technician cut

Milady's Art and Science of Nail Technology (Milady, 1992) states that nails ordinarily replace themselves every four months. The nail on the middle finger grows fastest, while the nail on the thumb grows slowest.

them, no matter how winter-dry and ragged they become. They are vital to nail health. Regular therapeutic soaking and moisturizing will revive them. Trimming them, using chemical solvents, or pushing them back vigorously can cause ridges in the nails. If the cuticle is damaged, the once watertight space under the *nail fold* (the deep fold of skin at the base of the nail, where the nail root is embedded) becomes susceptible to moisture and thus a potential breeding ground for bacteria and yeast infections.

If you frequently suffer from cold fingers, your nails may need extra stimulation to encourage proper blood flow. A daily nail massage with a good oil blend or a weekly at-home buffing can help. If your budget allows, a weekly professional manicure, complete with hand massage, is an indulgence to enjoy. Skip the polish if you wish. In no time, you'll see 10 nails (and cuticles) in beautiful tip-top condition.

Your nails, like your hair and skin, are mirrors of your general state of health or lifestyle. A healthy nail is smooth or very finely ridged, softly glossy, and translucent pink. Nail disorders such as deep ridges or furrows, thickening, discoloration, dimples, or slow growth can be indicative of systemic problems that could include malnutrition or illness or can result from excessive contact with dry air, water, soap, or chemicals. Even tools of the nail technician's trade — polishes, removers, artificial nails, nippers, scissors, brushes, and orangewood sticks — if improperly used or unsanitary, can physically harm nails or transmit bacteria and fungus.

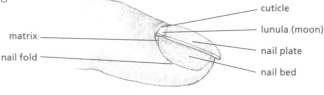

Parts of the fingernail

Skin Sense

Joel Gerson explains in *Milady's Standard Textbook for Professional Estheticians* (Thomson Learning, 1999) that "Blood and lymph supply nourishment to the skin . . . In the subcutaneous tissue are found networks of arteries and lymphatics that send their smaller branches to hair papillae, hair follicles, and skin glands." In short, all this physiology means that your skin is alive, and in order to keep your skin, hair, and nails looking their best and running at peak performance, you need to give them what they need to survive and thrive.

To insure a lifetime of healthy, vibrant good looks and an energetic body, you should observe what I call the seven lifestyle keys: daily cleansing, maximal nutrition intake, regular consumption of pure water, regular elimination of internal and external toxic buildup, daily movement, moderate exposure to sunlight, and sound sleep.

Step 1. Care for Your Skin Daily

Because your skin is constantly excreting wastes and shedding dead skin debris (sounds awful, but it's true), daily cleansing is a beauty must. All that's required is a mild, natural cleanser designed for your skin type (see What's My Skin Type?, below). If you wear foundation, powder, blush, or waterproof face and eye makeup, it's absolutely imperative that you remove this layer before going to sleep in order to avoid the possibility of clogged pores, blocked tear ducts, blackheads, and potential acne. Even if you don't wear makeup, it's a good idea to wash your face prior to bedtime, as the natural sebum on the surface of your skin readily attracts atmospheric pollutants and dirt like a magnet.

Speaking of dirt, here's a reminder: A telephone, whether personal or (especially) public, is usually filthy. This convenient communication device transmits a huge quantity of germs, dirt, and excess oil to your cheek, jawline, and mouth. Always clean your cell phone and land line at least twice a week using a good antibacterial cleanser or simple soap solution. And as your mother no doubt told you, always remember to wash your hands and keep them away from your face and mouth!

If you perspire a great deal in your line of work or if you exercise heavily, rinse off and massage your body with a coarse towel, then body brush (see page 36) or loofah before retiring to remove salt and dead-skin buildup.

What's My Skin Type?

Accurately assessing and caring for your skin type is key to having skin that is irresistible to touch and behold. Too many people treat their skin with the wrong products, and consequently, instead of improving its condition, they actually worsen it. What's more, skin type can change with the seasons, personal environment, health, and lifestyle. Yours may be different today than it was even a few months ago. It's important to know your *current* skin type in order to care for your skin in the best way.

Your skin probably falls into one of the following skin type categories, though some people may overlap two categories. Whether you lie in one classification or bridge two, though, it's important to assess your skin honestly and not judge what you have.

In each category you'll find ingredient and formula suggestions for recipes and methods of care. If you run across a particular ingredient or term that you don't understand (and you probably will), please see the index at the back of this book for all page references to that item. You'll be able to find an explanation or a formula recipe in no time. Also remember that in chapter 2, you'll find descriptions and explanations for all the ingredients used in the recipes in this book.

Normal or Balanced Skin

CHARACTERISTICS: This skin is neither too oily nor too dry. It's usually free of blemishes, but may form blackheads. It may get a little oily in the T-zone (forehead, nose, and chin area) or in the upper-back region four to six hours after cleansing, depending on humidity and temperature. The pores are normal in size. The entire body may suffer from surface dehydration (lack of moisture) in very cold weather. Normal skin is a balanced skin functioning as it should and is everyone's desired type.

CARE RECOMMENDATIONS: Use a mild soap as a cleanser *if you must* (see On My Soapbox, page 25), but it's best to use a gentler, water-based, nonfoaming or lotion-type cleanser on both face and body. Finely ground oat, nut, or seed blends and milk or clay blends are simple nourishing cleansers as well. Follow facial cleansing with an application of an herbal hydrosol mist or an herbal vinegar or tea toner to refresh and further cleanse the skin. Lavender, rose, calendula, lady's mantle, German chamomile, or rosemary are great mild herb choices. The moisturizer you choose for both face and body should be a lightweight yet protective lotion designed to seal in moisture. An herbal elixir is a moisturizing option for the face. If skin is prone to a bit of oiliness, avoid anything too heavy.

"When you improve your appearance, you also boost your morale. And we all function better and are more comfortable when we know we have presented our best to our critical selves and to the world."

VIRGINIA CASTLETON, AUTHOR OF
The Handbook of Natural Beauty

SPECIAL INTENSIVE TREATMENTS: For the face, use a weekly moisturizing mask or pore-refining, oil-absorbing clay mask. You can decide which treatment will benefit your skin most in any particular week — remember that skin condition fluctuates! These masks can be used on the chest, upper back, and throat as well. Fruit-acid masks made from papaya, apple, pineapple, or raspberry pulp are best used once or twice weekly to gently exfoliate, minimize fine lines, and smooth the skin. A weekly herbal facial steam will help keep pores clean.

Oily Skin

CHARACTERISTICS: This skin has medium to large pores in the T-zone area and perhaps on the cheeks, shoulders, neck, chest, and back. Overactive sebaceous (oil) glands can give oily skin a shiny appearance within an hour after cleansing. This skin may or may not be prone to acne, but oftentimes has clogged pores. Makeup seems to disappear or "slide off" oily skin after a few hours. Heat and humidity tend to increase its sebum production, whereas cooler temperatures and lower humidity are a boon for oily complexions. Surface dehydration may occur in very cold, dry weather. A bonus: Because it is well lubricated, oily skin is not prone to fine lines and wrinkles.

CARE RECOMMENDATIONS: You can use a gentle bar or liquid soap for face and body, but it's best to use twice daily a water-based gel or a finely ground oat, nut, or seed cleanser or a milk- or clay-blend cleanser that does not dry out the skin's surface. If oily skin becomes dehydrated on the surface, it will tend to produce more oil to compensate, which is not what you want. Your goal is to remove excess oil without stripping the skin of its protective barrier. Learn to equate "squeaky clean" with "dried out."

Follow face cleansing with the application of a gentle, herbal vinegar or tea astringent such as yarrow, sage, lemon balm, thyme, lemongrass, rosemary, parsley, or peppermint in order to remove cleanser residue and reestablish proper pH level. If you

CHEMICAL EXPOSURE AND YOUR SKIN: A POTENTIAL HEALTH RISK

I wouldn't be doing my job as a holistic esthetician if I didn't at least mention the potential health risk of exposing your skin to chemicals. If your work environment or hobby requires you to breathe or handle petroleum-based grease, welding gases, metal polishes, industrial or residential paints, solvents, toxic fumes, construction adhesives, coal or concrete dust, synthetic fertilizers, herbicides, pesticides, or any other "poison," please be sure to wear an appropriate breathing apparatus or mask and protective clothing — including gloves — at all times.

These chemicals and other "everyday" substances such as toxic household cleanser ingredients, can leach into your bloodstream via your skin, resulting in heavy metal or toxic chemical poisoning. The side effects are not pleasant, and without submitting to a blood test, the symptoms you may experience (such as headaches, nausea, weight gain, joint inflammation, dizziness, heart palpitations, nervousness, shortness of breath, high blood pressure, acne, eczema, mysterious rashes, and so on.) will probably be diagnosed as another type of illness.

So protect yourself during exposure and be sure to cleanse your entire body regularly (and definitely before sleep).

also suffer from an oily body, brew enough astringent or tea to use as a finishing rinse before you get out of the shower. Feel free to apply your choice of oil-removing liquid to face or body as often as necessary throughout the day. This procedure will remove excess sebum but will not dry your skin.

Depending on the degree of skin oiliness, a moisturizer may not be necessary for face or body. Beneficial, however, is a light, hydrating herbal hydrosol mist such as lemon balm, rose geranium — sometimes listed in catalogs as "geranium, rose" or "geranium (rose)," rosemary, or rose to keep the skin of the face moist throughout the day. You can apply a light moisturizing lotion to your body as needed. For the face, use an herbal elixir specially formulated for oily skin, such as the Healing Thyme Elixir on page 201, to help normalize sebum production.

SPECIAL INTENSIVE TREATMENTS: Use a clay mask or exfoliating scrub twice a week to discourage formation of blackheads, reduce the appearance of enlarged pores, and minimize breakouts. Fruit-acid masks used twice a week will remove dead skin cell buildup, refine the skin's surface, and minimize pore size. All masks and scrubs that you use on your face can be used on the body as well. *Note:* Do *not* use a granular scrub of any kind on the face or body if you suffer from acne, eczema, psoriasis, poison plant irritation, or any other type of skin inflammation; scrubs can further aggravate the condition.

A weekly herbal facial steam using sage, rosemary, strawberry leaves, yarrow, peppermint, or other astringent herbs will aid in detoxing facial skin and increasing circulation. As an overnight spot-treatment for minor blemishes or more active pimples, combine a drop of clove, tea tree, thyme (chemotype *linalol*), or lavender essential oil with a bit of clay and water to form a paste and dab this directly on the spot to disinfect, absorb oil, and kill bacteria.

THE pH FACTOR

You've seen it on everything from shampoos to soaps to skin-peeling creams, but what exactly is pH? The potential of hydrogen (pH) of a liquid refers to its degree of acidity or alkalinity, and the scale to measure it goes from 0 to 14, with the neutral point being 7, plus or minus a fraction of a point. Anything below a 7 on the pH scale is regarded as acid. Anything above a 7 is regarded as alkaline. When normal and balanced, your skin is typically mildly acidic, with a pH averaging between 5 and 6.

Most shampoos and especially bar soaps have a pH between 8 and 11 — quite alkaline, while most toners, astringents, and face splashes have a pH between 4.5 and 6, more on the skin-loving acid side.

Your skin maintains a healthy pH by forming an *acid mantle* from the combined secretions of your sweat and oil glands. Applying toners or astringents appropriate for your skin type (after using a mildly alkaline liquid cleanser or highly alkaline soap) returns your skin to its proper pH. Such products help prevent bacterial penetration and also help prevent the flaking, dryness, and tightness that can come from using soap-based cleansers. Diluted herbal vinegar, lemon water, various herb teas, and hydrosols are ideal for restoring a balanced skin pH.

Dry Skin

CHARACTERISTICS: This skin lacks natural oil and moisture, the basic requirements for a healthy glow. It may appear flaky or scaly and feel rough-textured, tight, or dry throughout the day. Dry skin has small pores and feels taut almost immediately after cleansing. It develops lines and wrinkles more rapidly than any other skin type and tends to age prematurely. Dry skin loves warm temperatures and humidity, but the winter can be a real challenge. Cold temperatures and winter air rob the skin of moisture, making it prone to irritation, sensitivity, redness, and chapping.

CARE RECOMMENDATIONS: You must avoid soap on your face and body at all costs. It's much too drying! Instead, use a moisturizing lotion or creamy cleanser; a finely ground oat, nut, or seed, cleanser; or a whole-milk cleanser.

For toning and hydrating, use a classic rosewater and glycerin lotion. Additionally, herbal teas such as German chamomile, calendula, fennel, lavender, lemon balm, marsh mallow root, and comfrey root applied to the face make excellent soothing toners. These gentle teas also make good after-bath splashes to hydrate dry and possibly sensitive skin. A quick spritz of chamomile, neroli, or lavender herbal hydrosol mist makes a great choice to alleviate thirsty skin any time of the day.

Never forget to moisturize the face and body. Use a rich cream or lotion that provides a barrier against dehydration and keeps moisture in the skin. You can also use an herbal facial elixir designed especially for the needs of dry or sensitive skin. In winter, underneath my moisturizer, I use Repair and Restore Elixir on page 202. When you've lived through a number of arid, cold, moisture-sapping New England winters, you quickly learn to *layer* moisturizers, much as you layer clothing — the more layers, the more protection from the biting cold.

SPECIAL INTENSIVE TREATMENTS: If you like to bathe in the tub, you can cleanse your body with a small, drawstring bath bag filled with ground oatmeal. Once wet, the oat flour covers your skin with moisturizing and soothing oat milk.

A mucilaginous fennel seed, marsh mallow root, or comfrey root facial steam once a week helps to hydrate the skin and cleanse the pores. Use a moisturizing mask once or twice a week as needed. For gentle facial exfoliation, try a weekly yogurt or fruit-acid mask made from apple or raspberry pulp. At least a couple of times per week, using a light touch, exfoliate your entire body (sans face) with a sugar, oat, nut, or seed scrub to remove buildup of dead skin cells. This is necessary to promote the absorption of your moisturizer; otherwise, all of the product's moisture remains on the surface of the skin and you'll wonder why it's not doing its job. The nightly use of an emollient eye cream or thin application of your favorite base oil moisturizes the delicate tissue in this area, which is prone to premature wrinkling.

Combination Skin

CHARACTERISTICS: If your face has two or three skin types, you have combination skin. It may be oily through the T-zone, where most of the oil glands are, and normal to dry toward the cheeks and sides of the face. In combination skin, the T-zone generally has enlarged pores and visible blackheads and may be prone to minor breakouts or even acne, while the cheeks and sides of the face and neck may feel normal and balanced or dry and tight, with possible surface flakiness.

This skin type is seasonally aggravated. In winter, the oily areas tend to normalize, while the dry areas feel parched. When heat and humidity rise, the T-zone increases its sebum production and the dry areas usually normalize.

CARE RECOMMENDATIONS: Combination skin is usually sensitive. *Always* treat it with TLC. Use products that regulate and normalize the sebum production for the entire face and upper body. Cleanse with a gentle, water-based, nonfoaming or lotion-type cleanser. Finely ground oat, nut, seed, milk, or clay blends are also nourishing cleansers. With combination skin, the skin of the body — with the exception of the chest and upper back, which are occasionally oily — is usually normal. If you want to use soap as your body cleanser, try a nonirritating, clear glycerin type or liquid castile designed for an infant's delicate skin.

For toning, a mild herbal vinegar infused with German chamomile, lavender, rosemary, fennel, roses, comfrey root, or calendula helps to control excess oil and hydrate dry areas. Any one of these herbs can be made into a tea and applied as a facial toner or used as a body splash immediately after showering or bathing. Rose, lavender, neroli, rosemary, lemon balm, and chamomile hydrosols are great hydrating mists to have on hand during the day to prevent surface dehydration. One of my favorite pore-tightening and skin-softening toner blends for combination skin is a combination of four parts yarrow tea mixed with one part vegetable glycerin.

For moisturizing the face, try an herbal elixir. Make one for oily skin (to use in the warmer months) and one for dry skin (to use in the colder months). If you feel the need for more intense moisturizing, apply a light- to medium-weight lotion to the driest areas only. For the body, a light lotion is all you need unless you live or work in an arid environment.

SPECIAL INTENSIVE TREATMENTS: Regular exfoliation of the skin on both the face and oilier parts of the body using a nonabrasive mask removes dead skin buildup to keep pores open. Once or twice a week, use a pore-refining clay, yogurt, oatmeal, or fruit-acid mask — try the Papaya No-More-Pores Double Mask Treatment on pages 152–153 — to improve this skin's texture and minimize pore size. You can also enjoy a facial steam once each week using an herb of your choice such as lemon balm, peppermint,

On My Soapbox

Most soaps on the market today are highly alkaline and chock full of chemicals and artificial fragrances and can strip your skin of its protective oils, leaving it dry, tight, flaky, itchy, and prone to eczema. Consequently, it's generally not recommended to use soap on the face and neck unless you have extremely oily skin, and even in this instance, it should be used only in the warmest months.

I'm well aware that there are a number of people who swear by soap. You've used it all your life, you may say — every day, from head to toe, and even to wash your hair. That squeaky-clean feeling can make you feel *ultra fresh!* And because I know that old habits are hard to break, I won't insist that you give up your favorite bubbly bar. I do suggest, however, that you use the gentlest of soaps, such as those tolerated by sensitive skin: a super-fatted, low-lathering bar; a goat milk–based bar; a clear glycerin bar or liquid soap; or a nonirritating, liquid castile soap designed for infants.

Remember that regardless of your skin type, the most effective and nurturing way to cleanse your skin is to use a gel, lotion, or creamy cleanser; a finely ground oat, nut, or seed cleanser; or a milk- or clay-blend cleanser. If you wear foundation makeup or work in a greasy environment, you can follow this with a second cleansing using a glycerin soap made specifically for the face.

rosemary, thyme, or lemon peel to improve the tendency of combination skin toward sluggish circulation.

Sensitive Skin

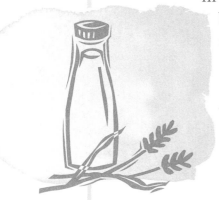

CHARACTERISTICS: *Environmentally reactive* is how I like to refer to skin that is sensitive. It tends to overreact to outside forces such as commonly used skin care products, sunlight, and changes in temperature and humidity. This skin type easily blushes, sunburns, develops rashes, and becomes irritated. Especially when more mature, it typically displays *couperose* conditions — that is, it's characterized by dilated or expanded capillaries. A diffused redness, or *erythema*, is generally concentrated on the nose and cheeks. If not treated extremely gently, sensitive skin will simply appear "unhappy" or "unsettled."

Crisp, dry winter air can further upset already irritated, sensitive skin, leaving it drier and more prone to disturbances. Summer's heat, humidity, and increased exposure to sunlight can also wreak havoc, leading to itchy, blotchy skin, possible blemishes, and general ruddiness.

CARE RECOMMENDATIONS: Follow all recommendations for dry skin, above, unless skin is normal to oily, in which case use a lightweight to medium-weight moisturizer for both face and body. Cleansing only with an *ultra soft* cloth — no terry towels, facial loofah sponges, or brushes on this delicate skin!

SPECIAL INTENSIVE TREATMENTS: Follow recommendations for dry skin, above. When choosing any treatment product or ingredient, *gentle, nonabrasive, and fragrance-free or fragrance-tolerable* are the key words on which to focus.

Mature Skin

CHARACTERISTICS: Skin can generally be referred to as being mature when you can detect an apparent loss of tone and the skin exhibits a crepelike texture: It's saggy and loose with many fine lines and at least a few shallow or even deep wrinkles. Most of the time such skin is found in people over age fifty, as part of the natural aging process, but I've seen mature skin on individuals as young as their early forties, and, for the lucky few, these signs don't reveal themselves until the early sixties. Good genes, plenty of natural oil in the skin, a healthy lifestyle and sound nutrition, and proper consistent skin care all determine when or to what extent mature skin appears.

This skin type tends to be dry but can be normal or slightly oily in the T-zone, especially if the skin was oily earlier on. If you are over fifty and have oily skin, however, consider it a boon — you'll wrinkle later than your friends. Mature skin is generally more comfortable in warmer climates with higher humidity. In cooler, more arid surroundings, it ages faster and tends to suffer from additional dryness. Such skin may also have hyperpigmentation (age spots, freckles, or liver spots), depending on an individual's history of sun exposure, smoking, and alcohol consumption.

CARE RECOMMENDATIONS: Moisture retention is key to preventing the rapid increase in fine lines and wrinkle depth, so it's important not to use drying soap, especially on the face. Remember that the collagen and elastin matrix within the dermis layer depends on constant hydration to maintain plumpness. For facial cleansing, use a gentle lotion or cream cleanser once or twice a day if you have dry skin or a lighter lotion cleanser if your skin is normal to oily. Finely ground oats, milk or dairy cream, and fat-rich sunflower seeds make super-moisturizing cleansers for

GOT DRY SKIN? MAKE OIL YOUR BEST FRIEND

I've found a lasting solution to my very dry body skin in the winter months: Every day I thoroughly massage my favorite body oil into my skin immediately after showering. Try this: Roughly towel dry first, leaving your skin slightly damp, then apply the oil. I top it off with a layer of body lotion or cream. This double treatment acts as a protective barrier: It prevents the moisture you already have in your skin from evaporating and locks in the moisture you've just received from the shower or bath. This procedure works so well that I rarely have winter-dry, itchy skin anymore!

face or body. Use a clear glycerin or super-fatted soap on the body only, unless you have normal-to-dry skin.

My favorite toners for mature skin are a classic rosewater and glycerin lotion and a lavender, German or Roman chamomile, rose geranium, neroli, or rose tea or hydrosol mist. Try using a soothing rosewater and glycerin lotion as a body splash on occasion, especially when your skin is very dry.

For moisturizing both face and body, depending upon the degree of dryness and the season, use an easily absorbed nutrient-rich lotion or cream. An herbal elixir containing carrot seed essential oil and rose hip seed base oil, key ingredients in Repair and Restore Elixir (page 202) and valued for their highly regenerative and vitalizing properties, can be used as your only facial moisturizer or as a first layer followed by lotion or cream if your skin is extra-thirsty. Avoid rose hip seed oil if your skin is oily; it can lead to breakouts.

SPECIAL INTENSIVE TREATMENTS: To minimize the appearance of fine lines and wrinkles, fade age spots, and help maintain a smooth, refined appearance, twice weekly use a fruit-acid facial mask made from papaya, raspberry, strawberry, or pineapple puree (unless you have sensitive skin). A honey mask or moisturizing facial mask deeply hydrates mature skin tissue and can be used daily. Enjoy a fennel seed, lavender, or calendula facial steam once a week to hydrate, cleanse impurities from the pores, and increase circulation.

Use a rich body oil following each shower or bath to seal in moisture and keep skin supple. Eye cream should be applied as part of your daily skin care ritual. Because skin naturally thins and produces less oil as you age, by the time you reach your fifties, the already paper-thin skin surrounding your eyes has become even more translucent, drier, and wrinkle-prone. For youthful-looking eyes, don't forget these hints: don't squint, and invest in a snazzy pair of quality sunglasses!

Environmentally Damaged Skin

CHARACTERISTICS: This skin type, with its premature lines, wrinkles, hyperpigmentation (freckles and age spots), ruddiness, rough texture, and uneven skin coloration, may begin to rear its ugly head somewhere around age 35. Much to the shock of those who have it, it often takes on the characteristics of mature skin. Environmentally damaged skin is *lifestyle reflective.* Those who tend to have this skin type include smokers, coffee and cola drinkers, consumers of large amounts of alcohol, routine recreational drug users, ocean-sport enthusiasts, sun worshippers, mountain climbers, long-distance walkers or runners, or any lover of sports that take place in the most extreme outdoor climates. These people generally have skin that has been repeatedly severely dehydrated, and it may be impossible to return it to its former healthy, radiant suppleness. Collagen and elastin, the proteins located in the dermis layer, have lost their elasticity and flexibility.

Individuals with healthy, naturally fair, thin, dry skin that easily becomes environmentally damaged over time, tend to suffer from painful, papery, parched skin that bleeds and tears easily when elderly. Be sure to take extra precautions when exposing yourself to the elements or engaging in harmful lifestyle choices.

Environmentally damaged skin might have been oily or normal in its youth, but it's almost always at least normal-to-dry if not very dry after the age of 40.

CARE RECOMMENDATIONS: Because such skin is frequently sensitive and dry, read the sections on sensitive skin and dry skin for information on those types.

For environmentally damaged skin, each season brings its own challenges. Always remember that your skin needs deep hydration and constant sun protection. For the face and body, a nonirritating, mild, water-based lotion or creamy cleanser fortified with skin nourishing oils such as jojoba, hazelnut, extra-virgin olive, or macadamia deep-cleans and feeds your skin. Finely ground oat, nut, and seed cleansers and milk-based cleansers are gentle skin foods that encourage softness and soothe irritation. If the skin on your body is dry, please avoid soap.

For toning, *mild* and *nondrying* are key words. A lavender, lemon balm, chamomile, or neroli hydrosol refreshes and removes any excess cleanser from the face. *Skin quenching tip:* Never leave home without a spritzer bottle of purified water or your favorite hydrosol. Throughout the day, every hour if desired, spray a light mist on your face. This keeps your makeup fresh and your skin from becoming flaky, dull, uncomfortable, and drab-looking.

For moisturizing, a lotion or cream enhanced with rose hip seed, coconut, macadamia, extra-virgin olive, or jojoba oil helps to feed, rejuvenate, tone, and support cell membrane functions within the skin of both the face and the body. An herbal facial elixir with carrot seed, rosemary (chemotype *verbenon*), neroli, green myrtle, or helichrysum essential oil helps stimulate new cell generation and encourage a brighter appearance.

SPECIAL INTENSIVE TREATMENTS: See recommendations for dry skin.

Step 2. Maximize Your Nutrition

Pizza; French fries; iceberg lettuce; lifeless, unripe tomatoes; jelly beans; hamburgers; chips; processed frozen dinners; ketchup: What does this group of foods provide? White processed flour, fatty meat and cheese, excess sodium, trans-fatty acids, preservatives, white sugar, minimal fiber, and artificial coloring. A diet of these foods is void of all nutrient value and is a recipe for health and beauty disaster. Yet these are some of the most commonly eaten "foods" in the American diet today. The four veggies on the list — iceberg lettuce, French fries, unripe tomatoes, and ketchup — describe the narrow variety of produce consumed by many children and adults in any given week. Sad, isn't it?

We are often overfed and undernourished. The average American these days is overweight and out of breath, certainly doesn't look his or her vibrant best, and is aging prematurely — inside and out. Most Americans appear and feel older than their years, proving "You are what you eat."

If you belong to this group, you'll continue to suffer from lack of energy and vitality and a variety of aches, pains, and illnesses. What's more, what we eat directly affects how we look. At some point, your outward appearance will reflect this insufficient nutrition, with lifeless hair, brittle nails, and pallid, problematic, toneless skin. Remember that *if you always do what you've always done, you'll always get what you've always got.*

The quickest and least expensive way to change your looks and feel better mentally and physically is to clean up your diet. You can make effective improvements easily.

Much of the mass-produced food today is not raised or made with an eye toward your maximum fuel potential, but instead for corporate profits. Intensive farming practices and poor soil management produce foods that tend to lack taste and nutrients. Add synthetic chemical fertilizers, pesticides, herbicides, and genetic engineering to the mix, and you've got additional woes.

Your diet should consist of foods that are high in complex carbohydrates, low in fat, high in fiber, and moderate in lean protein. You should consume daily a wide variety of foods in their whole, natural, preferably organic, unprocessed state, including several servings each of fresh fruits, vegetables, whole grains, and beans; a few tablespoons of fresh, raw nuts and seeds; and a little extra-virgin olive, flaxseed, or unrefined coconut oil.

Consume eggs from certified, organically raised chickens in protein shakes and fruit smoothies or cook them any way you like. You can even enjoy them on a daily basis or several times a week if you avoid other animal sources of protein. (*Note:* If you have or are prone to high cholesterol, please check with your physician before eating eggs this frequently, even if you abstain from eating meat.)

Meat, poultry, and seafood eaters should limit their consumption to three to four ounces per day (about the size of a deck of cards) and try to buy only organic, free-range chickens or turkeys; wild, deep-sea fish (such as salmon, cod, mackerel and haddock) and shellfish; and grass-fed beef or pork from cows and pigs raised without hormones, steroids, and antibiotics. Alternative animal sources of protein such as lamb, venison, goat, and buffalo are frequently untainted by chemicals. Remember to avoid *excess* consumption of animal proteins; they're often high in fat and totally void of fiber.

You can also meet protein requirements with vegetarian choices such as soybean products (tofu, tempeh, soy burgers, and so on), rice and pea protein powders, nut butters, seeds, sprout breads, bean sprouts, seaweed, and bean and grain combinations.

A wholesome, balanced diet containing these products nourishes the inner body and is reflected on the outside.

Whole-Food Supplements

Along with a whole-foods diet, nutritional supplements also have their benefits to your well being. No matter how balanced you think your diet is, virtually everyone has a deficiency of one nutrient or another. Supplements help fill in the nutritional gaps so that you look and feel your best — giving you the appearance of youth (or actually prolonging your youth) from the inside out.

While many professionals believe differently, I believe that the most effective supplements are derived from whole, real foods (as opposed to being entirely synthetic). I take my three favorite supplements on a daily basis. Combined, they contain all of the specific nutrients that help combat aging, nourish skin, hair, and nails, and promote well-being.

"Not only does beauty fade, but it leaves a record upon the face as to what became of it."

ELBERT HUBBARD, AMERICAN PHILOSOPHER, WRITER, AND PUBLISHER

GREEN DRINK BLEND. Every morning, I toss a handful of frozen raspberries, strawberries, mango chunks, or a frozen banana into the blender, then add a cup or more of soy or rice milk, a dollop of plain goat yogurt, and two tablespoons of an organically produced, green plant powder. The one I use contains "powerhouse plants" including chlorella, a single-celled green algae; blue-green algae; barley grass; wheat grass; and alfalfa.

When choosing a green-plant powder blend, make sure the product label states that the ingredients were organically grown and were processed rapidly immediately after harvesting to preserve the live enzymes and vitamins they contain. The grasses taste the way a freshly mowed lawn smells — sweet and green. The blend is also available in easy-to-swallow capsules.

OPCS (OLIGOMERIC PROANTHOCYANIDINS). Yup, it's a tongue-twister, but here's a short explanation: OPCs are becoming recognized as one of the most potent categories of antioxidants (which act as *anti-aging* or *youthifying* agents). They fight the free radicals that cause oxidation, the process responsible for the rusting of metal, the browning of a cut apple, or the appearance of brown age spots on your body. OPCs are present only in plants and have blue-green, yellow, red, and purple pigments.

An OPC supplement is available in liquid or powdered form at any good health food store and often includes: red wine, purple and red grapes, prunes, raisins, blueberries, blackberries, red bilberries, lingonberries, raspberries, spinach, kale, currants, rose hips, turmeric, ginger, pine bark, grape seeds, green tea, gingko leaf, hawthorn leaf, and oregano. It's recommended that you include many of these foods in your daily diet. An added bonus: Liquid OPC formulations are usually quite delicious, tasting like fruit juice.

A MIX OF RAW SUNFLOWER AND PUMPKIN SEEDS. Mix equal parts of raw sunflower seeds and raw pumpkin seeds (sometimes called pepitas) in a plastic container or bag and carry this tasty, crunchy treat with you as a healthy fast-food snack or toss it in your daily salad in lieu of white-bread croutons. For a zestier taste, sprinkle a bit of your favorite salt-free seasoning on the mix.

These seeds have essential fats and substantial amounts of iron and zinc. Raw, unprocessed, unheated omega-3 and omega-6 fatty acids may be two of the most powerful tools in the anti-wrinkle arsenal. Fat preserves your skin's suppleness and youthful sheen. Raw fats also have potent anti-inflammatory properties, promoting heart health and relief of pain.

Another option: consume a tablespoon or two of fresh flax-seed, extra-virgin olive, fish, or unrefined coconut oil.

Step 3. Drink the Elixir of Youth and Health — Water

Earlier, I stressed the importance of water's role in keeping your skin plump and hydrated and nutrients flowing to your newly forming skin, hair, and nail cells.

What's the difference between a prune and a plum, an ocean marsh and the Sahara Desert, and the smooth skin of a teenager and the sagging and wrinkled skin of a ninety-year-old? Water — the simple, pure, essence of life that makes up approximately 70 percent of each of us. It's one of the most important and most abundant inorganic substances in the human body. In fact, it is by far the most abundant material in all tissues, with the exception of tooth enamel and bone. Your blood, the "living highway," is primarily composed of water.

The body literally can't move or function, inside or out, without water. You can't bend or stretch, blink, yawn, smile, jump up and down, poop, breathe, sweat, or even think without water lubricating every part of your physical being or assisting transport of vital substances, nutrients, and oxygen toward and away from your body's parts and systems.

You cannot be beautiful, energetic, and healthy without sufficient water intake. With ample moisture, the elastin and collagen matrix in the dermis layer of your skin stays plump, and a hydrated, well-fed hair or nail root produces a shiny, strong hair shaft or nail. Conversely, a dehydrated person ages prematurely and is exhausted.

In addition to pure water, fresh (preferably not canned or pasteurized) fruit and vegetable juices are also a source of this fluid. Part of your daily water intake can also come from raw

> "Beauty never forgets its essence, even if we — and our world — have. Given any opportunity, beauty will reestablish itself."
>
> KAT JAMES, AUTHOR OF
> *The Truth about Beauty*

whole fruits and veggies, which are composed primarily of this fluid. Try to consume at least six glasses a day for internal and external health and well-being. If you hate drinking plain water, try adding a squeeze of lime, lemon, or orange juice to the glass. A splash of cranberry or cherry juice concentrate added to water also makes a deliciously tangy treat.

Step 4. Detox Your Skin with Regular Elimination, Inside and Out

Simply stated, your skin serves as the interface between your inner and outer worlds. To keep both worlds detoxified and comfortably functioning, regular removal of bodily wastes must take place via internal elimination and the routine removal of such deposits from the top layer of your skin.

Internal Flushing: Fiber and Water

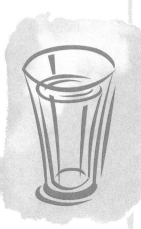

What goes in must go out. Ample fluid intake combined with a fiber-filled diet keeps the digestive system moving right along, eliminating toxins via your colon and preventing them from surfacing on your skin as rashes and blemishes. Impurities that aren't disposed of in a timely manner via the kidneys, liver, lungs, and large intestine will find an alternate exit — which is why the skin is sometimes referred to as the "third kidney." Being "regular" contributes to physical comfort, does a world of good for your mood, and keeps the skin clear and radiant.

External Brushing: Beauty and the Body Brush

One of my favorite health-promoting rituals, which I enjoy every morning just prior to showering, is *body brushing* or *skin brushing* (sometimes also referred to as *dry brushing* because it's performed on dry skin).

Over the course of an average day your skin eliminates more than a pound of waste, including perspiration. In fact, about one third of all the body's impurities are excreted this way. If your skin is not carrying out normal elimination due to basic neglect of hygiene; illness; dry skin buildup; medication side effects; repeated application of mineral oil–based, pore-clogging body lotions or waterproof chemical sunscreens; or nutritional deficiencies; then your kidneys, large intestine, liver, and lungs may be operating on a subpar level. Therefore, anything you can do to improve skin function improves the function of the other elimination organs.

Body brushing — a health-enhancing, age-old tradition undergoing a renaissance in today's wellness spas — takes only about five minutes before showering or bathing. It works by stimulating the sebaceous glands, thereby encouraging natural moisturizing of your skin; removing the top layer of dead cells, leading to significant exfoliation and skin that's polished and silky; improving circulation and increasing blood flow to the surface of the body; and activating the entire lymphatic system, thereby aiding in natural detoxification.

Another benefit that I've noticed is improved tone in the "jiggle-prone" parts of my body: upper arms and inner thighs. In addition, my complexion is rosier, body lotions and oils penetrate more easily, and — a bonus I didn't expect — it doesn't take me thirty minutes to wake up in the morning, like it used to! For me, body brushing is equivalent to a shot of espresso. Not bad for a five-minute beauty treatment!

Perform this treatment daily. It will take your skin a while to get used to it. Here's how: Using a medium-soft, natural-fiber brush the size of your palm, preferably with a handle, simply brush your entire body — don't skip any areas except your face (and breasts, if you're a woman) — for five minutes or so, depending on body size.

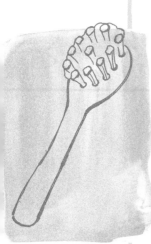

Do not brush hard — you'll have to start very gently at first (even more so if you have very sensitive skin) and work your way up to more vigorous brushing. *Never* scrub, however; your skin is not the tub! Always remember to brush toward your heart as much as possible. Begin brushing your hands, including the area in between the fingers, then work upward to your arms, underarms, neck, chest, and upper back. Next, move on to each leg, beginning with the feet and working upward toward the groin, buttocks, lower back, and sides. End at your stomach, using a clockwise spiral motion to brush this area. That's it!

You'll feel wonderfully invigorated when you're finished, and your skin will glow. If you're just beginning, your skin may be a bit red immediately afterward, but as it adjusts and becomes firmer, only a pinkish tinge (depending on your pigmentation) will remain for about five minutes until circulation calms. If your skin remains red or pink for a longer period, then either the brush bristles are too firm or you're brushing way too hard. *Note:* Avoid dry brushing altogether if your skin is sunburned, windburned, rashy, or otherwise irritated.

As a final step, jump in the tub or shower and bathe as usual. All of the dead skin you just loosened will be washed away. Afterward, be sure to pat — not rub — your skin until it's almost dry, and then apply your favorite body oil or moisturizer.

It's a good idea to wash your body brush with mild soap and water every week or so to keep it free of odor and skin debris.

Step 5. Keep Moving to Look and Feel Your Best

Lead your body in the right direction, and the health of the skin follows. Regular physical exercise increases lymphatic flow and circulation, improves digestion, stimulates your metabolic

Good Food and Good Looks: Make the Connection

If you were born in the 1950s or 1960s and followed the fashion world at all, you'll probably recognize the name Carol Alt. Now in her late forties, Alt was one of the first official super-models. She's also an accomplished actress and author of *Eating in the Raw* (Clarkson Potter, 2004), an eye-opening treatise on the role a raw-food diet can play in lifelong health, good looks, and prolonged youth.

As a *raw foodist*, Alt believes in eating only foods that have not been cooked or chemically altered by heat, which can destroy many heat-sensitive vitamins and alter the protein structure of animal products. The raw-food diet includes fruit and vegetable salads, juices, smoothies, nuts, seeds, sprouts, raw dairy, sushi, raw shellfish, and steak tartar. According to Alt, consuming a completely raw-food diet has done a world of good for her overall health, skin quality, and vitality — all of which make her look much younger than her years.

While a 100 percent raw-food diet is not for everyone, eating this way from time to time can make you feel great. There are important elements of a raw-food diet that should be incorporated into your daily nutrition: large quantities of preferably organic, fresh, raw fruits and vegetables; sprouted grains; and nuts and seeds. These will go a long way toward improving the way you both look and feel.

fire and the process of waste removal from the internal organs and skin, and delivers a surge of oxygen to your body, invigorating every organ and allowing your skin to take on a radiance. Without regular exercise, your maximum skin health and beauty cannot be revealed. The body will actually deliver nutrient-carrying blood and oxygen to the other organs first before it takes the care of the extremities — your skin, hair, and nails.

Another fact: Daily exercise is vital to your emotional well-being. It can energize you in the morning or help you unwind after work, eliminating or reducing the stresses of the day. Exercise acts as a natural antidepressant.

In order to promote my cardiovascular health, flexibility, core strength, and muscle tone, I take a brisk 45- to 60-minute walk almost every day, usually with my 90-pound Irish setter leading the way, followed by 15 minutes of gentle, deep stretches or yoga poses. On alternate days, I add a 20- to 30-minute series of strength-building exercises with free-weights, plus military push-ups, squats, lunges, abdominal work, and a stint on my cable-style weight machine. A firm, toned body exhibits the shape of youth and health.

Try to exercise in the fresh air and sunshine as often as possible and vigorously enough so that you work up a good sweat. Sweating cools your skin and eliminates waste through your pores. If you don't like to walk, then choose whatever you enjoy: biking, jogging, swimming, Pilates, aerobics classes, tennis, or even rollerblading. There really is an activity for everyone. It's up to you to find it and stick with it, or choose several and alternate to prevent boredom. If you are over the age of 35, have been inactive for a period of time, or have any health problems or concerns, be sure to get your health professional's okay before beginning any exercise program.

Step 6. Give Yourself Some Exposure: A Little Sun Is a Good Thing

We've become a sunphobic society. Yet all living things — plants, animals, and people — need at least a *little* sunshine in order to survive and thrive. Certainly, *overexposure* to the sun is the single most damaging factor to your skin. It's not just a sunburn but also a suntan (and the associated skin dehydration) that represent damage to your skin, and that damage is cumulative over a lifetime.

Yet sunshine feels good on your skin and helps your body absorb calcium by causing your skin to produce part of the vitamin D complex that strengthens bones. Sun exposure also aids in healing eczema, acne, psoriasis, and poison ivy rash; helps reduce stress and blood pressure; balances hormone levels; and increases the body's production of feel-good serotonin.

Thirty to 45 minutes of daily unprotected exposure to sunlight in the early morning before 9:00 AM or very late afternoon, after 4:30 or 5:00 PM, can help preserve your sanity and the health of your bones and skin. If you live in the north, where sunshine is sometimes limited in the winter and temperatures can be quite cold, try to expose your face and hands for at least 15 minutes daily. Many health professionals have observed a rise in the occurrence of osteoporosis, spontaneous fractures of the small bones of the feet, vitamin D deficiencies, skin diseases, mood imbalances, and SAD (seasonal affective disorder) not only in this country, but also globally because our lives are increasingly sedentary and spent indoors, with long car commutes between work and home. Increasing our sun exposure slightly can affect the incidence of these conditions.

"Green is the prime color of the world, and that from which its loveliness arises."

PEDRO CALDERÓN DE LA BARCA,
SPANISH DRAMATIST AND POET

Sun exposure is a subject of much debate, however, and if your health professional or dermatologist has advised that you avoid the sun at all costs due to various health concerns, then your body will require other sources of vitamin D. This essential nutrient can be found in egg yolks; fish liver oil; vitamin D–supplemented cow, soy, or rice milk; organ meats; salmon; sardines; and herring.

While brief, unprotected sun exposure may be beneficial, when you intend to spend a longer period of time in the sun, it's important to apply sunscreen *prior* to exposure, wear protective clothing, and use "common sun sense": Don't stay in the sun for hours on end with no protection of any kind or without reapplying sunscreen regularly, and avoid exposure during the middle of the day, when the sun's rays are at their strongest. These strategies will help prevent premature aging, uneven skin tone and blotching, and exposure that may cause skin cancer.

Though it's important to wear sunscreen, the chemicals in most commercial products can be very irritating to many wearers, especially those who exercise outdoors. Sunscreens can sting if they drip into your eyes or nose and can cause the development of skin rashes when their chemical base mixes with sweat. Natural sunscreens, such as those containing titanium dioxide and zinc oxide, provide a physical, sun-reflective barrier; offer a relatively high SPF; and greatly reduce or eliminate irritation. Natural oil blends containing jojoba, neem, or sesame oil are beneficial skin emollients and conditioners that also provide a low natural SPF. See chapter 4 for some natural sunscreen recipes.

As for tanning, if you must have a deep, golden tan, then try a self-tanning lotion or cream available in drug and department stores. Follow the directions, do a patch test, and take the time to apply an even layer. The results are quite realistic if the lotion is applied correctly.

Observing "common sun sense" beginning in your teen years or early twenties can virtually stop the visible aging clock. But at any age, it's never too late to begin to care for your skin and health in the sun.

DON'T FORGET COMMON SUN SENSE

Last July, after one of my best friends and I completed an exhausting five-mile power walk through the 95°F, baking hot, Texas hill country (slathered in natural sunscreen, of course), we laughed at how bedraggled and red-faced we looked. My friend then offered this quote: "In life's journey to the grave, we shouldn't intend to arrive safely in a pretty and well-preserved body; rather, we should skid in broadside, thoroughly used up and totally worn out, loudly proclaiming, 'Wow! What a ride!'"

After walking in the south Texas heat, that's exactly how we both felt: used up, covered in sweat, and totally worn out — but also happy, relaxed, and stress-free. By far the most important accomplishment of our walk, though, was catching up on the important gossip of the week! Exercising with a friend is a terrific time for socializing.

Outdoor exercise and sports can be fun, and at times, even exhilarating — but remember: It doesn't have to come at the expense of your skin's health. So if you're an avid outdoorswoman or outdoorsman, keep Mother Nature's sun, heat, salt, drying wind, cold, or arid climate at bay by always drinking plenty of water and wearing your "shield" of moisturizers, natural sunscreens, protective clothing, and sunglasses!

Step 7. Seek Deep, Restful Sleep

Did you get a good night's sleep last night? If you're like most people, the answer is probably no. Sleep is often the first thing we sacrifice due to work commitments, children's demands, lifestyle choices, or the activity of today's hustle-and-bustle world. In fact, sleep doesn't get much attention until it's sorely missing. The solution: Instead of thinking of sleep as a luxury or as something you can put off and catch up on later, think of it as an essential nutrient, just like vitamin C or water. Nighttime is the right time for renewal, and those prized hours when you sleep are the optimal time for your body's repair and rejuvenation.

Human growth hormone, which aids in the repair of damaged cells, including those of the skin, hair, and nails, is produced while you sleep. When you're sleep-deprived, your body struggles to maintain itself mentally and physically. Lack of sleep shows up as dark under-eye circles; haggard, sallow skin; puffy eyes; dull hair; lackluster nails; low energy level; weakened immunity; mental meltdowns; depression; irregular appetite; and lack of sexual interest. Sleep deprivation can also trigger the release of *cortisol,* your stress hormone. Overproduction of cortisol ages your skin and contributes to unmistakable signs of fatigue. You can't put your best face forward when running on empty!

A solid night of shut-eye is often referred to as *beauty sleep* or *beauty rest* because it's one of the best (and least expensive) beauty secrets of models and celebrities or anyone who depends on physical appearance for his or her livelihood. You can spend scads of money on the latest eye cream or trendy spa treatments, but a good dose of sleep is the most effective beauty and well-being treatment of all.

TWO

The Natural Apothecary

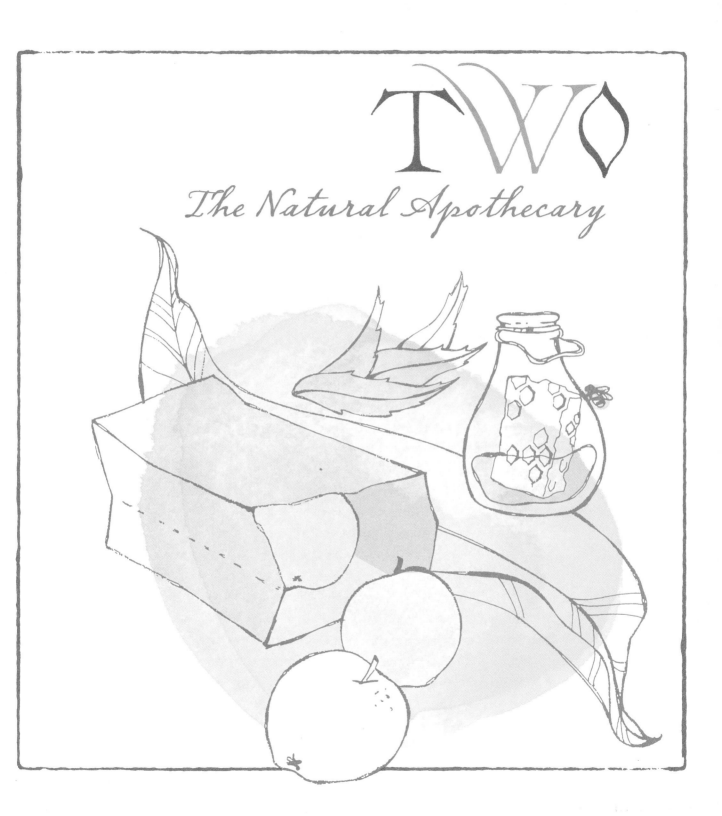

This chapter details the ingredients called for in the personal care recipes that begin in chapter 4. For your convenience, the Ingredient Dictionary (see page 57) lists substitutes, when applicable, that can be used when an ingredient called for in a particular recipe is unavailable.

Where do you find these ingredients? Your local health food store or whole foods grocer is the first place to check for beeswax, cocoa and shea butters, essential oils, base or carrier oils, raw seeds and nuts, organic herbs, and grains. If you have no luck there or live in a rural area where availability may be limited, try the local pharmacy or cosmetic supply house. They may carry a handful of the items you need, including storage containers, or may be able to order them for you. The Yellow Pages are also an excellent place to find ingredients. Look under "Botanicals," "Herbs," "Nurseries," "Garden Centers," "Health Food Stores" and "Natural Food Stores," "Restaurant Supplies," "Perfumes," "Pharmacies," "Spices," and "Oils."

If you have a green thumb, you can grow many of the herbs from seed (depending upon your climate) or from herb plants available at your local garden center. You can also forage for herbs in the wild. If you decide to go this route, however, be sure to purchase a good illustrated herb book (preferably with color photos) and educate yourself while hiking through the woods and meadows. A wild plant identification class offered by a local herb school, county extension service, or adult education program would be well worth the time and expense.

I purchase most of my ingredients from mail-order catalogs or Internet sources. Sometimes, while traveling in the northeast, I get lucky and stumble across a small, New England farm that can provide organically grown herbs or oats for soothing facial scrubs and bath bags. Fresh raw honey and beeswax direct from the apiary is a real luxury that I like to include in lip balms, body butters, and creams. When driving around the countryside, always keep an eye out for purveyors of farm specialties that could be used in personal care recipes. A fresh ingredient is a first-rate ingredient! For a listing of tried and trusted ingredient suppliers, see Resources, page 358.

An Ingredient Primer

There are many individual ingredients listed here that will be quite familiar to you, such as baking soda, sea salt, pineapple, honey, and lemon, and my brief description of each one will be sufficient for your complete understanding of their use in personal care recipes. There are four broad categories of personal-care ingredients, however, that require an in-depth introduction: base oils; essential oils; herbs; and meal blends made from seeds, nuts, and oats. In the following pages you'll come to understand the specific terminology, quality, storage requirements, harvesting, or preparation techniques for the ingredients in each of these categories. Before you purchase any ingredients and start blending, grinding, mixing, and melting, take a few minutes and educate yourself. Remember: A knowledgeable consumer makes the wisest choices and the highest-quality handmade body care products.

Base Oils

Often referred to as *carrier oils,* these are derived from seeds, nuts, beans, vegetables, and fruits and, as their name implies, are used as a base to which essential oils, solid fats, thickeners, watery liquids, or herbs and spices are added when making herb-infused oils, lotions, salves, balms, elixirs, and creams. Base oils can also be used alone or in combination with other base oils when creating massage and bath oils, hair and skin conditioners, or makeup-removing products.

The best base oils for personal care recipes are those that have been organically grown, naturally extracted, and minimally

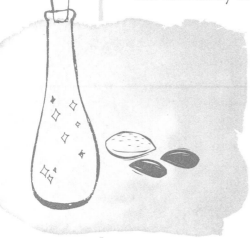

processed. The key words to look for on the label are *unrefined, expeller pressed,* or *cold-pressed.* These oils have not been exposed to the extremely high temperatures, chemical extraction procedures, bleaching, or deodorizing that can destroy or alter natural aromas, flavors, antioxidant properties, beneficial vitamins, and trace minerals. These gently processed oils are produced by mechanically pressing nuts, seeds, beans, fruits, or vegetables, then straining any resulting debris. Some heat is naturally generated during the pressing, but it's not so high that it destroys the vital nutrients, taste, and aroma of the oil. As compared to their highly processed, refined cousins, be aware that organic, unrefined oils are slightly darker in color, deeper in aroma, truer to taste (if eaten), and exceptionally higher in essential fatty acids. They may also have a cloudy appearance at times.

These oils — with the exception of jojoba, neem, calophyllum, and castor oils — are also highly recommended for use in cooking and salad dressings; they have a better flavor and higher nutritional value than conventionally processed oils commonly found in supermarkets.

Note that due to lack of processing and superior freshness, an unrefined base oil — with the exception of jojoba, neem, extravirgin olive, and coconut oils — has a short shelf life and tends to become rancid if stored at room temperature for more than six to eight months, especially in warm weather. These oils should thus be refrigerated and used within one year. If the oil you are using has a strong or "off" smell (with the exception of extra-virgin olive, neem, calophyllum, sesame or coconut oils; these have naturally strong fragrances), then it's probably old and rancid. Purchase base oils through reputable retailers with a high turnover of inventory. Always check the expiration date on the bottle and never hesitate to return the oil if it's bad.

At times, the terms *slip and slide* are used to describe the way an oil or oil-based product glides onto the skin. A particular oil that has a *nice slip* or *slides well* smoothies or flows onto the skin effortlessly under mild hand pressure — that is, the oil or product is neither sticky nor too rapidly absorbed. An oil with these properties is perfect to use as a body or face massage oil. Organic almond and soybean oils are excellent massage base oils because of their thinner texture. I also like jojoba oil, an excellent balancing body oil, because it's chemically similar to human sebum, leaving desert-dry skin velvety soft and aiding in normalizing oily skin.

Essential Oils

Essential oils are primarily extracted by steam distillation, with the exception of citrus oils, which are generally cold-pressed from the rind. A newer method of extraction is called *carbon dioxide (CO2) extraction*. Essential oils from tree resins such as frankincense and myrrh and from calendula blossoms are sometimes extracted in this manner. Another method used is *solvent extraction*, and the resulting oils are referred to as *absolutes*. Jasmine, rose, and mimosa are common absolutes and are recommended for perfumery and fragrance use only and not for skin and body care products. (Due to the synthetics remaining in the end product, this type of oil is not considered of therapeutic grade.)

The following are a few examples of the plant parts from which particular oils are derived:

PLANT PARTS USED FOR ESSENTIAL OILS

spearmint and peppermint..............leaves and stems
chamomile, neroli, and lavender.......flowers
cinnamon ....bark or leaves
lemon, lime, and orange................rind
pine and spruce ....needles
juniper....................................berries
cedar ....wood
gingerroot and vetiver ....root
fennel and anise ....seeds

Unlike a base oil, an essential oil, despite its name, is not actually an oil because it does not contain fatty acids and is not prone to rancidity. Essential oils *do not* dissolve in water or aloe vera juice and dissolve only a little in vinegar. They *do* mix very well in base oils and break down relatively well in rubbing alcohol or common "drinkable" alcohols such as vodka, brandy, gin, rum, whiskey, and so forth.

I consider essential oils the *life force* or *soul* of the plant. They embody the plant's precious, aromatic hormones and chemical compounds that can regenerate and oxygenate the skin. Essential oils are important to include in therapeutic personal care formulations because, due to their minute molecular structure, they easily penetrate into the dermis to nourish, rejuvenate, and revitalize skin cells, unlike many of the heavier ingredients in face and body care products, such as base oils, waxes, and thickeners, which remain primarily on the skin's surface or penetrate only slightly beneath it.

ESSENTIAL OIL TIPS

Essential oils are highly concentrated natural products and must be used with caution. Only one precious drop of rose otto essential oil is produced from approximately thirty rosebuds — but not all flowers and herbs are that stingy with their essential oil. Always educate yourself about the properties and contraindications surrounding each essential oil before you use it. To determine potential allergic reactions to a specific oil, try this test: Combine 1 or 2 drops of the essential oil with ½ to 1 teaspoon of base oil in a small bowl. Apply a dab on the underside of your wrist, inside your upper arm, behind your ear, or behind your knee and wait 12 to 24 hours. If no irritation develops, the oil is safe to use.

Essential oils are so highly concentrated that few may be used *neat* (undiluted) on the skin: lavender, tea tree, German chamomile, rose, sandalwood, and geranium (rose geranium). Always dilute an essential oil in a base oil unless you know it's safe to use neat.

If, while working with an essential oil, you rub or splash the oil into your eyes or nose — which can cause excruciating pain — immediately flush the affected area with an unscented, bland fatty oil such as almond, olive, corn, soybean, peanut, or generic vegetable oil. Whole milk makes a substitute for the fatty oil in an emergency. Using plain water does not help; essential oils are attracted to fats alone. Should the pain continue or should severe headache develop, seek prompt medical attention.

Essential oils retain their healing properties for 5 to 10 years if properly stored in a dark, dry, cool place, and some actually improve with age. The exception to this is citrus oils: They will remain potent for only 6 to 12 months unless refrigerated, and if refrigerated, may last up to two years or so if not frequently opened. Because they can be harmful if ingested, it is advisable to store essential oils out of reach of children and pets.

Herbs

Herbs have been collected by all civilizations. They have been prized for their medicinal, nutritional, flavorful, fragrant, cleansing, and skin-pampering properties and have been revered for use in magical, ritual, and spiritual ceremonies.

As you try your hand at some of the recipes here and come across an herb that really intrigues you, my advice is to further educate yourself. Look up the plant in two or three herb books; study all its possible uses, both current and historical; learn its charms, growth habits, harvesting and storage requirements, any contraindications, and the various uses that current herbalists recommend. This additional information will augment your direct experience.

All herbs, flowers, leaves, seeds, barks, berries, and roots called for in the recipes in this book are relatively common, easy to find, and used in *dried* form unless otherwise specified. If you have access to freshly grown herbs, then you may want to dry the herbs yourself. See the following instructions for harvesting, drying, and storage. Recently dried herbs have a wonderful, just-picked aroma and vital nutrients that are at their peak — they'll simply make your products all the more delightful.

Tips for Harvesting and Drying Herbs

You may be surprised by how easy it is to dry many of the herbs from your garden. No matter which technique you choose, it's best to dry them as soon as they're picked so that their beneficial properties are not diminished. Here are other key points to keep in mind:

- Always use a sharp knife when harvesting. Gather herbs in early to mid-morning, just after any evening dew has had a chance to dry but before the sun becomes too hot.

- Harvest flowers such as roses, calendula, chamomile, or lavender as soon as the bud is mature and well-formed or the flower has just opened. A bud or bloom that is past its prime does not have the fragrance, color, or bounty of volatile oils that a fresher specimen has.
- Be careful to harvest herbs that are free of insects and disease and have not been treated with pesticides. Herbs for harvesting should be relatively dirt-free, but if they're dusty or if you've gathered them from a roadside where they've been exposed to wafting debris, you can quickly rinse them in cool water and immediately pat them dry with a paper towel. Be sure to handle them gently; the leaves and flowers can bruise easily. To remove all dirt from harvested roots, gently scrub and then vigorously rinse them.
- Avoid overdrying herbs; it can diminish their valuable properties.
- Dried herbs should be stored in a cool, moisture-free place away from direct sunlight. Zip-seal plastic bags, glass jars, plastic tubs, or metal tins make great storage containers.

Hang Drying Herbs

To dry your herbs by hanging, simply gather together in a bundle 5 to 10 stems of a single herb and secure the bundle using a string, rubber bands, or a clothespin around the stems. Hang bundles upside down in a well-ventilated, dimly lit area where the humidity is low. The ideal temperature for drying is between 65°F and 85°F. Leave plenty of room between bundles to insure good air circulation and to keep scents from mingling. Because many herbs look similar when dried, you may find it helpful to label your bundles.

Herbs can take anywhere from four days to three weeks or

more to dry completely, depending upon weather conditions and the thickness of leaves, stems, and flowers. Roots and seeds take the longest due to their high moisture content. When dried herbs are ready for storage, leaves will be brittle but not so dry as to shatter easily; flower petals and buds will feel dry and semicrisp or powdery; roots will be hard or ever-so-slightly pliable; and berries, bark, and seeds will be very hard and dry.

Screen Drying Herbs

Many herbs can also be successfully dried on metal or nonmetal screens or tightly stretched netting. The open mesh allows air to flow freely around the plant and quickly evaporate its moisture.

To prepare herbs for screen drying, separate the leaves, flowers, buds, roots, berries, barks, and seed heads from the stems and spread them in a single layer over the screen. Leave enough space between all plant parts to allow for good air circulation. Drying times vary from a few days to a few weeks, depending on humidity levels. If you're setting up screens outside, they should be in a partly shady area. Cover the plant material with a single layer of cheesecloth or another screen to keep out airborne debris, feathers, or pet dander and other dirt or dust. Keep an eye on the weather, too — you don't want rain, drizzle, or fog to ruin your harvest. Soggy, moldy herbs are fodder for the compost heap.

Nut, Seed, and Grain Meal Blends

I always have a fresh supply of the following three "skin food" staples in my freezer: almonds, sunflower seeds, and regular or old-fashioned oatmeal. No crafter of handmade personal care products should be without these body beautifiers. All three should be organically grown, if possible, and used in their raw form — never toasted, roasted, or salted. When a recipe calls for a particular meal, simply follow the instructions below and add the appropriate quantity to the formula you are making. *Note:* Measurements are approximate due to size variations of the ingredients.

BUYER BE AWARE

Essential oil production is a labor-intensive and expensive project. It takes approximately five hundred pounds of rosemary to produce one pound of oil. Jasmine absolute, one of the most expensive essential oils (it retails for $300 to $600 per ounce) requires approximately 8 million handpicked blossoms, harvested before sunrise, to produce just over two pounds of oil. A high-quality oil is expensive, but it's worth it. Unfortunately, some oils are poor quality, so be aware of the distinguishing features of a quality product.

- Look for the terms *g & a* (genuine and authentic), *vintage,* or *organic* on the label, or ask for therapeutic or pharmaceutical grade oils, which have been steam-distilled at low temperatures. You'll pay more for these, but you'll be sure to get a pure, effective product.
- Essential oils are highly volatile and evaporate quickly. Place a drop on a sheet of plain paper, spread it around, and then leave it for 5 to 10 hours. A real essential oil will evaporate and leave either no stain or a very small one. A vegetable oil will leave a greasy stain much like that made by potato chips kept in a paper bag.
- Vegetable oils have a greasy feel; essential oils do not. Rub a little vegetable oil between your fingers and notice how slippery it is. An essential oil may initially feel a bit greasy, but it's absorbed quickly or feels more like water. If the essential oil feels like vegetable oil, it has probably been diluted.

Almond Meal

To make ½ cup of almond meal, in a blender, small food processor, or coffee grinder, grind (in 5- to 10-second pulses) approximately 50 to 75 medium to large raw almonds until the consistency is that of finely grated Parmesan cheese. Be careful not to overblend. Due to almonds' high fat content, it's very easy to unintentionally end up with almond butter, especially if you're using a small grinder that generates lots of heat.

Sunflower Seed Meal

To make ½ cup of sunflower seed meal, in a blender, small food processor, or coffee grinder, grind ⅔ to ¾ cup of large, hulled seeds until the consistency is that of finely grated Parmesan cheese.

Ground Oatmeal

To make ½ cup of ground oatmeal, in a blender, small food processor, or coffee grinder, grind ¾ to 1 cup of regular or old-fashioned oats until the consistency is somewhere between fine and coarse flour.

ETHICAL WILD-HARVESTING

None of the herbs listed in this book are on the endangered list, but nonetheless, a rule of thumb to remember when harvesting herbs in the wild (after first asking the landowner for his or her permission to trespass) is never to overharvest an area. Pick only what you need at one time, leaving plenty of root stock in the ground and fully mature, adult plants remaining so that a new generation of seedlings will emerge during the next growing season. With the resurgence in popularity of herbs, overharvesting of wild plants is becoming a global problem leading to the scarcity of formerly common plants. Don't contribute to this loss!

The Ingredient Dictionary

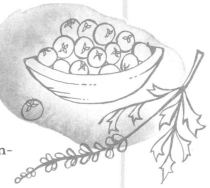

Here is a comprehensive listing of ingredients called for in the handmade personal care recipes found in chapters 4–9. Included in each description is valuable information about what each ingredient is and what it will do to beautify and pamper your body. Get to know these ingredients; they are your tools for renewed radiance, vibrance, and well-being. Use this compendium as a reference guide as you create and concoct your lotions, cleansers and scrubs, body balms and butters, sensual treats, and intimate helpers.

Almond, Meal (*Prunus dulcis*)

PARTS USED: Raw almonds, ground into a meal

COSMETIC PROPERTIES AND USES: High in skin-pampering emollients (softening fats or lipids), almond meal can be used as a body or facial scrub and mask base to gently exfoliate surface dry skin. Good for all skin types. With regular use, it acts as a gentle bleaching agent to help even skin tone.

POSSIBLE SUBSTITUTES: Ground sunflower seed meal

CONTRAINDICATIONS: To avoid further skin irritation, do not use as a scrub if skin is acneic, sensitive, sunburned, or windburned.

Almond Oil, Sweet (*Prunus dulcis*)

COSMETIC PROPERTIES AND USES: Derived from the ripened, pressed kernel, this is an all-purpose, pale golden, nutritious, lightweight or medium-weight base oil that can be used in a wide range of products from lotions and massage oils to body butters. It has a high fatty acid content and penetrates well. Recommended for all skin types, especially dry, inflamed, or itchy skin.

POSSIBLE SUBSTITUTES: Apricot, hazelnut, sunflower, or soybean oil

Aloe *(Aloe vera)*

PARTS USED: Fresh gel from leaves or fresh, bottled juice. (Commercial juice should be at least 99 percent pure with less than 1 percent added oxidation and mold inhibitors.)

COSMETIC PROPERTIES AND USES: Mildly astringent aloe is soothing to oily, normal, and normal-to-dry skin. It relieves the irritation from sunburn, minor skin burns and rashes, and insect bites and helps restore the skin's natural pH.

Anise Seed *(Pimpinella anisum)*

PARTS USED: Essential oil

COSMETIC PROPERTIES AND USES: This spicy, sweet, warming, and stimulating essential oil is traditionally used to aid digestion and as a flavoring agent. It can be used to flavor and scent lip balms, body balms, and personal lubricants.

POSSIBLE SUBSTITUTES: Fennel seed essential oil

CONTRAINDICATIONS: Avoid if pregnant or epileptic. May be a potential skin irritant.

Apple *(Pyrus malus)*

PARTS USED: Flesh as fresh, raw fruit puree or applesauce

COSMETIC PROPERTIES AND USES: The juice of the apple contains malic acid (as does apple cider vinegar) and acts as a mild astringent and gentle, nonabrasive exfoliant. It's soothing and nourishing for acneic and sensitive skin.

Apple Cider Vinegar, Raw

COSMETIC PROPERTIES AND USES: Containing malic acid, it can be used as a gentle, nonabrasive, exfoliating astringent (always diluted with water) for all skin types except very dry. It soothes and relieves itchy, scaly skin and restores the skin and scalp's natural pH. It also helps control dandruff and remove styling-product buildup when used as a hair rinse.

CONTRAINDICATIONS: Avoid use on sensitive, sunburned, or windburned skin.

Apricot Kernel Oil (*Prunus armeniaca*)

COSMETIC PROPERTIES AND USES: A base oil derived from the kernel of the apricot, it has properties similar to almond oil, though it's a bit lighter in weight, texture, and color and is odorless. This oil is excellent for softening the delicate skin around the eye and on the throat. It's recommended for use in eye creams and facial elixirs for oily-to-normal and mature skin due to its skin tightening ability and slight astringent quality.

POSSIBLE SUBSTITUTES: Almond, hazelnut, or soybean

Arrowroot (*Maranta arundinacea*)

COSMETIC PROPERTIES AND USES: Arrowroot powder is made by grinding the thick, dried arrowroot rhizomes into a starchy, white, bland powder similar to cornstarch. Use as a base for body and foot powders.

POSSIBLE SUBSTITUTES: Cornstarch

Avocado (*Persea americana*)

PARTS USED: Pulp, base oil

COSMETIC PROPERTIES AND USES: This full-bodied, light-green base oil is derived from the fatty pulp and seed of the fruit. Both oil and fruit pulp are rich in nutritive and conditioning components such as vitamins A, B_1, B_2, D, and E that are especially helpful to dry, dull skin and hair. Due to its heavy emollient texture, the oil takes a bit longer than other base oils to penetrate the top layer of skin. It's especially good to use in outdoor sport creams or after-bath massage oils. Avocado oil leaves a protective barrier on the skin to help prevent moisture evaporation.

POSSIBLE SUBSTITUTES: Sunflower or olive oil

HOW TO MAKE AN HERBAL INFUSION

Herbal infusions (or herbal teas, as they're most commonly referred to by nonherbalists) are frequently used in the recipes here as an ingredient in face and body splashes, facial toners, hair rinses, lotions, creams, and bath additives. To make a cup of herb tea, pour 1 cup of boiling water over 1 heaping teaspoon of dried herb or 2 heaping teaspoons of fresh herb. Cover, steep 5 to 10 minutes (or overnight if you want a strong brew), and strain. Cool and use as directed.

Baking Soda (*Sodium Bicarbonate*)

COSMETIC PROPERTIES AND USES: This white, odorless, alkaline, salty-tasting powder has skin-soothing and softening properties. It relieves the pain and itch of bee stings and the itch from rashes, deodorizes feet and underarms, and softens bath water.

Banana (*Musa paradisiaca* var. *sapientum*)

PARTS USED: Pulp

COSMETIC PROPERTIES AND USES: This nourishing and moisturizing fruit is used for its gentle, nonabrasive exfoliation and skin-tightening action in face and hand masks. It's good for all skin types, especially normal and dry.

Basil, Sweet (*Ocimum basilicum*)

PARTS USED: Essential oil

COSMETIC PROPERTIES AND USES: This essential oil has a fresh, spicy-sweet, "green" scent that's very uplifting. It conditions hair and scalp and is used in formulas to stimulate hair growth.

POSSIBLE SUBSTITUTES: Rosemary essential oil is much less expensive and nearly as effective when used to promote hair growth.

CONTRAINDICATIONS: Avoid if pregnant or epileptic.

Beeswax

COSMETIC PROPERTIES AND USES: Pure, unrefined, unbleached, filtered or unfiltered beeswax is used as a thickener in creams, lotions, salves, butters, and balms. It adds a sweet, honeylike fragrance and golden color to products.

POSSIBLE SUBSTITUTES: Vegetable emulsifying wax, but this wax has been refined and does not have the same alluring qualities as beeswax. Always try to find the real thing!

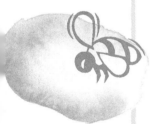

Bergamot (*Citrus bergamia*)

PARTS USED: Essential oil

COSMETIC PROPERTIES AND USES: Cold-pressed from the peel, bergamot, used to flavor Earl Grey tea, has a full, round, floral and citrus fragrance that refreshes, balances, and helps to ease anxiety, nervous tension, and depression. Use this essential oil for sleep and dream balms.

POSSIBLE SUBSTITUTES: Sweet orange essential oil, but it has a much lighter, fruitier fragrance than bergamot. Children seem to like sweet orange better, however.

CONTRAINDICATIONS: Avoid use if pregnant or epileptic. May be photo-sensitizing and a potential skin irritant if skin is sensitive.

Bhringaraj *(Eclipta alba)*

PARTS USED: Leaves

COSMETIC PROPERTIES AND USES: This is commonly used in Ayurvedic hair and scalp remedies, both applied externally and consumed as a supplement. (Ayurveda, meaning "the science of life," is one of the world's oldest systems of health care based on the integrative study of body, mind, and soul. It originated in India over five thousand years ago.) Bhringaraj is known in India for its abilities to promote hair growth and help prevent premature graying and is also used to calm the mind. It's included here in soapless herbal hair shampoo recipes for its gentle, stimulating properties.

Birch, Sweet *(Betula lenta)*

PARTS USED: Essential oil

COSMETIC PROPERTIES AND USES: This essential oil has a fresh, minty, sharp aroma identical to wintergreen. It can be used in anti-inflammatory, antispasmodic balms to help soothe sore muscles, painful joints, sprains, and arthritis, as well as in decongesting sinus balms.

POSSIBLE SUBSTITUTES: Wintergreen essential oil

CONTRAINDICATIONS: Avoid if pregnant or epileptic. May be a potential skin irritant.

Blackberry *(Rubus villosus)*

PARTS USED: Leaves

COSMETIC PROPERTIES AND USES: Use as a gentle astringent ingredient for oily and normal skin.

POSSIBLE SUBSTITUTES: Strawberry, sage, or raspberry leaves

Borax *(Sodium Borate)*

COSMETIC PROPERTIES AND USES: A white, crystalline mineral powder commonly available in the laundry aisle of grocery stores, this acts as a binder and texturizer; when combined with beeswax, oil, and water, it aids in the formation of a stable emulsion. It also acts as a whitener, weak antiseptic, and natural preservative. Borax is frequently combined with sea salts, Epsom salt, and baking soda in making natural bath salts. Like baking soda, it softens hard water.

CONTRAINDICATIONS: To avoid creating a cloud of potentially irritating mineral dust, gently scoop (versus pour) borax from its container when adding to recipe.

Brahmi *(Centella asiatica)*

PARTS USED: Leaves

COSMETIC PROPERTIES AND USES: Also known as *gotu kola,* this herb is commonly used in Ayurvedic hair and scalp remedies both as an external wash and as a supplement. Brahmi is believed to revitalize the nerves and brain, strengthen memory, and improve concentration. It can be used in soapless herbal hair shampoos as a gentle, stimulating astringent to aid in removing excess oil.

POSSIBLE SUBSTITUTES: Peppermint or rosemary leaves (external use only)

Cajeput *(Melaleuca cajeputi)*

PARTS USED: Essential oil

COSMETIC PROPERTIES AND USES: Cajeput has an uplifting, penetrating, camphorous aroma similar to tea tree essential oil. It acts as a respiratory stimulant, helping to decongest blocked sinuses and tight lungs. Use in making sinus and cold and flu balms and oils.

POSSIBLE SUBSTITUTES: Tea tree essential oil

CONTRAINDICATIONS: May be a potential skin irritant if skin is sensitive.

Calendula *(Calendula officinalis)*

PARTS USED: Flower petals, essential oil (CO_2 extract)

COSMETIC PROPERTIES AND USES: Orange calendula flowers are known for their calming, anti-inflammatory, and skin-healing properties. Slightly astringent and antiseptic, the herb and essential oil can be used in lotions, creams, elixirs, and balms for all skin types — especially for skin that is sensitive, environmentally damaged, acneic, irritated, or chapped. It's excellent in children's formulas. An infusion of the flowers can be used as a brightening rinse for blond or red hair.

POSSIBLE SUBSTITUTES: German chamomile essential oil and flowers

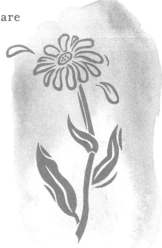

Calophyllum Oil *(Calophyllum inophyllum)*

COSMETIC PROPERTIES AND USES: This rich, brown-green base oil is also known as tamanu or foraha oil. Derived from the ripened seeds of a native Tahitian tree, it has a sweet, earthy fragrance reminiscent of buttercream frosting or Kahlua. It's analgesic, antibacterial, and anti-inflammatory. Use it in oil blends specifically formulated to help fade scars; heal burns; and soothe chapped skin, eczema, and psoriasis. It's a perfect choice for environmentally damaged, mature, or very dry skin.

Cardamom *(Elettaria cardamomum)*

PARTS USED: Essential oil

COSMETIC PROPERTIES AND USES: This oil has a sweet, spicy, woody, citrus fragrance derived from the cardamom pod. Use this stimulating and warming oil as an exotic perfume addition to milk bath, bath oil, and massage oil recipes. It blends well with other essential oils such as neroli, orange, cedar, and ylang ylang. For an intoxicating romantic combination, mix it with rose and vanilla essential oils.

Carrot Seed (*Daucus carota*)

PARTS USED: **Essential oil**

COSMETIC PROPERTIES AND USES: A clear, pale-yellow essential oil, this has a warm, dry, woody, earthy aroma. It aids in restoring elasticity to sagging, wrinkled, or sun-damaged skin, but is excellent for all skin types. Combine it with rose hip seed base oil when making facial elixirs and under-eye moisturizing treatments.

CONTRAINDICATIONS: Avoid use if pregnant or epileptic. May be photosensitizing and a potential skin irritant if skin is sensitive.

Castile Soap, Liquid

COSMETIC PROPERTIES AND USES: This gentle, olive oil–based soap can be used to bathe the entire body or can be used as an herbal shampoo base. If you have oily skin, this is the soap to choose.

POSSIBLE SUBSTITUTES: Your favorite synthetic-free, low-lathering shampoo base or liquid glycerin soap will work as well as castile soap.

CONTRAINDICATIONS: Avoid use on dry skin, scalp, and hair.

Castor Oil (*Ricinus communis*)

COSMETIC PROPERTIES AND USES: This clear to slightly yellow, shiny, viscous base oil is processed from the seeds of an annual shrub. It's highly emollient and provides staying power and shine to lip balm and lip gloss recipes. (It's the primary oil in most creamy and glossy lipsticks on the commercial market.) It's particularly good for softening rough, dry heels, knees, and elbows and patches of eczema and psoriasis. When applied to nails, it imparts a protective shield against exposure to drying detergents, hot water, and winter-dry air.

Catnip (*Nepeta cataria*)

PARTS USED: **Essential oil**

COSMETIC PROPERTIES AND USES: The active component in catnip oil (*nepetalactone*) is reported to be more effective at repelling mosquitoes than DEET, the toxic chemical ingredient included in many commercially available insect repellents. The fragrance is pungent, woody, and minty and has sedative, calming effects on people (opposite the catnip plant's effects on your feline friends). *Note:* This oil is toxic as an inhalant for cats. Please store it in a safe area away from pets.

CONTRAINDICATIONS: Avoid if pregnant or epileptic.

Cedarwood *(Juniperus virginiana)*

PARTS USED: Essential oil

COSMETIC PROPERTIES AND USES: This essential oil has a classic, stimulating, cedar aroma, yet is a bit smoother and more full-bodied. It's a skin-friendly additive to natural insect repellent formulas.

Chamomile, German *(Matricaria recutita)*

PARTS USED: Flowers, essential oil

COSMETIC PROPERTIES AND USES: This deep-blue, floral-scented essential oil is high in *chamazulene* and *alpha bisabolol* (chemical components known for calming and healing). Use it for treating sensitive or inflamed skin: Dermatitis, eczema, psoriasis, and active acne respond well to this healer. Use the pretty yellow flowers in skin teas or toners, lotions, and creams for normal or dry skin. Chamomile infusion is also used as a subtle lightening and brightening rinse for blond or light brown hair. Blend dried powdered flowers into body powder recipes for both babies and adults.

POSSIBLE SUBSTITUTES: Moroccan Blue Chamomile *(Tannecetum annuum),* also called blue chamomile or blue tansy and *not* to be confused with *Tannecetum vulgare,* or common tansy, which is toxic.

Chamomile, Roman *(Anthemis nobilis)*

PARTS USED: Essential oil

COSMETIC PROPERTIES AND USES: This golden oil has mild antispasmodic, calming properties, but it's primarily used here in massage and body oils and creams for its sweet, applelike, floral fragrance. Its scent relaxes the mind and may help relieve anxiety. It blends well with other floral essential oils such as rose, ylang ylang, geranium, and neroli.

Cinnamon Bark (*Cinnamomum zeylanicum*)

PARTS USED: Powdered bark, essential oil

COSMETIC PROPERTIES AND USES: Use sharp, spicy, warming cinnamon powder (my favorite is Vietnamese) primarily to add fragrance to masks and face or body scrub recipes. It has antiseptic and antibacterial properties, but only in amounts so great that they'd be irritating to the skin and nasal passages. The essential oil can be used as a fragrance and flavoring in lip and edible body balms and in making flavored toothpicks, though it's very potent and will irritate sensitive skin and mucous membranes. Use with caution.

CONTRAINDICATIONS: Avoid getting cinnamon powder into eyes and mucous membranes — it may cause tearing, stinging, or sneezing. Avoid using essential oil if pregnant or epileptic.

Citronella (*Cymbopogon nardus*)

PARTS USED: Essential oil

COSMETIC PROPERTIES AND USES: This essential oil offers a tart, earthy, lemony aroma along with insecticidal, antispasmodic, antiseptic, and deodorant actions. It's classically used as a natural insect repellent added to candles, incense, and skin formulations.

CONTRAINDICATIONS: Avoid if pregnant or epileptic. May be a potential skin irritant.

Clay, Powdered: White, Green, and Red

COSMETIC PROPERTIES AND USES: Clay is derived from the ground and its formation is the result of hundreds of years of decay and compression of composting debris and rainwater. It's extremely mineral-rich, which is why it's so good for the skin. Various types can be used in creating masks, face and body cleansers, and body powders. When used in masks, it has remarkable absorbent powers. As it dries, it actually raises the temperature of the skin, encouraging toxin and excess sebum removal. Used as a face or body cleanser, it acts as a gentle exfoliant, leaving skin velvety smooth. In body powders, it helps keep the skin deodorized and moisture-free.

CONTRAINDICATIONS: Avoid clay-based masks if you have dry skin; they draw oil from the skin. A clay-based or clay- and grain-blend cleanser is fine, though, because it's immediately rinsed off instead of remaining on the skin to harden like a mask.

White Clay

Also referred to as cosmetic clay, this is a very mild, fine clay that's practically pure aluminum oxide with traces of zinc oxide. It's best suited for environmentally damaged, sensitive, mature, and delicate skin, unless very dry. It's so gentle that nearly anyone can use it.

Green Clay

This pale green clay (sometimes called French green clay), has a high concentration of chromium, nickel, and copper. It's best suited for oily and combination skin because it aids in reducing sebum production. It also works well on acneic skin, which often can't tolerate irritating chemical peels and harsh, granular exfoliants.

Red Clay

A rusty, medium-red color, it has a high iron, silica, magnesium, calcium, and potassium content and is best suited for cleansing and toning normal skin.

Clove Bud (*Eugenia caryophylatta*)

PARTS USED: Essential oil, whole cloves

COSMETIC PROPERTIES AND USES: This is spicy, warming, stimulating, and broadly antiseptic. Add whole cloves to men's aftershave recipes primarily for the fragrance. When diluted in a base oil, the essential oil acts on sore muscles and joints.

CONTRAINDICATIONS: Avoid if pregnant or epileptic. May be a potential skin irritant.

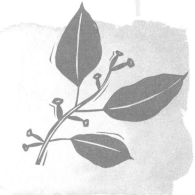

Cocoa Butter (*Theobroma cacao*)

COSMETIC PROPERTIES AND USES: Derived from the cocoa bean, this sweet, chocolate-fragranced, emollient butter is hard at room temperature but melts when applied to the skin. It lends a thick consistency to lotions, creams, body butters, balms, and salves. It's a wonderful addition to recipes for personal lubricants; after-sun care; and edible, flavored body balms. It tastes like a combination of vanilla beans and chocolate.

Coconut Oil (*Cocos nucifera*)

COSMETIC PROPERTIES AND USES: Use only organically grown, unrefined coconut oil. Its sweet, exotic fragrance and smooth flavor are reminiscent of a tropical paradise. Refined coconut oil is void of both sweet fragrance and flavor. Coconut oil is a highly emollient base oil derived from the fruit of the coconut palm and is solid at temperatures below 76°F. It's an excellent oil for all-over use, and some swear by it as the ultimate skin softener, hair conditioner, and after-sun treatment. Use this tasty, healing oil in lip balms; personal lubricants; edible, flavored body balms; body creams; lotions; or any oil-based skin product from which you desire a penetrating, softening effect.

Comfrey (*Symphytum officinale*)

PARTS USED: Root

COSMETIC PROPERTIES AND USES: Comfrey root infusion or tea is soothing, healing, mildly astringent, slightly mucilaginous, and emollient. Use the infusion as a gentle, hydrating toner for inflamed, sensitive, environmentally damaged, or dry skin. Make a strong, simmered brew, dip your clean fingers into the liquid, and notice how slippery and smooth it feels. Your skin will find this herb very comforting.

POSSIBLE SUBSTITUTES: Marsh mallow root

COCONUT TIDBITS

According to a *Skin Inc.* magazine article by Kate Hamilton, in Sanskrit, coconut is *kalpa vriksha,* meaning "the tree that provides all the necessities of life"; in Malay, it's called *pokok seribu guna,* "the tree of a thousand uses"; and in the Philippines, it's called simply "the tree of life." Early Spanish explorers called it coco, or "monkey face," because the three indentations on the furry fruit resemble the face of a monkey.

Cornmeal (*Zea mays*)

COSMETIC PROPERTIES AND USES: Cornmeal is a naturally abrasive exfoliant used in body and facial scrub recipes.

CONTRAINDICATIONS: Avoid use on acneic, inflamed, sensitive, sunburned, or windburned skin.

Cream, Dairy (*Light or Heavy*)

COSMETIC PROPERTIES AND USES: This fatty emollient is a superb additive (instead of water) for softening normal and dry skin when mixed with powdered face and body cleansers and scrub blends. It's also very soothing.

Cucumber (*Cucumis sativus*)

PARTS USED: Fresh, peeled slices and strained juice

COSMETIC PROPERTIES AND USES: Cucumber is mildly astringent and soothing and has a slight bleaching action that helps even skin tone.

Elder Flower (*Sambucus canadensis*)

PARTS USED: Flowers

COSMETIC PROPERTIES AND USES: The fragrant flowers make a soothing wash for both eye and skin irritations. Good for all skin types.

POSSIBLE SUBSTITUTES: Comfrey root

Epsom Salt (*Magnesium Sulfate*)

COSMETIC PROPERTIES AND USES: This salt relieves aches and pains and lactic acid buildup in overused muscles and is good for use in sore-muscle-soak recipes and bath salt blends. It's especially good for reviving dog-tired, achy feet.

CONTRAINDICATIONS: If pregnant or breast-feeding, consult a health professional before use. Avoid use on irritated, sensitive, abraded, sunburned, or windburned skin. May sting and further dehydrate already dry skin.

Eucalyptus (*Eucalyptus radiata*)

PARTS USED: **Essential oil**

COSMETIC PROPERTIES AND USES: **Also known as narrow-leaved peppermint eucalyptus, this essential oil has powerful antiviral and antiseptic capacities and can decongest and open sinuses. Cooling to the skin, it also helps relieve sore muscles and feet. Multiple varieties of eucalyptus are available; *E. globulus* is more common, but *E. radiata* is gentler.**

Fennel, Sweet (*Foeniculum vulgare*)

PARTS USED: **Seeds, essential oil**

COSMETIC PROPERTIES AND USES: **Add sweetly fragrant, licorice-like fennel seed to facial steam blends for its gentle, cleansing, soothing, and hydrating benefit to all skin types. A fennel-seed infusion makes an all-purpose toner or splash for everyone's skin. The seeds themselves can be chewed to freshen breath or added to men's aftershave blends for their slightly spicy, sweet aroma. Because it tends to deodorize, use the stimulating essential oil to fragrance foot scrubs and balms.**

POSSIBLE SUBSTITUTES: **Anise essential oil**

CONTRAINDICATIONS: **Avoid if pregnant or epileptic.**

Fir, Balsam (*Abies balsamea*)

PARTS USED: **Essential oil**

COSMETIC PROPERTIES AND USES: **This provides a stimulating, woody, "holiday" aroma used as a sinus decongestant and respiratory antiseptic. Because it helps relieve nervous tension and depression and is balancing to the psyche, use this oil in sleep-enhancing balms, chest rubs, and sinus balms. The fragrance seems to open the lungs and encourage deeper, fuller breathing.**

Frankincense (*Boswellia carterii*)

PARTS USED: **Essential oil (CO_2 extract)**

COSMETIC PROPERTIES AND USES: **The sweet, heavy fragrance of this oil traditionally used for perfumery and in incense blends is reported to reduce anxiety and tension by slowing and deepening breathing. It's derived from dried plant resin. Also use it to rejuvenate tired, sagging** skin and accelerate the healing of skin blemishes and small wounds. Frankincense is a wonderful ingredient in facial elixirs or oil blends for acneic, environmentally damaged, or mature skin.

Geranium, Rose (*Pelargonium graveolens* or *Pelargonium* x *asperum*)

PARTS USED: **Essential oil**

COSMETIC PROPERTIES AND USES: Sometimes you'll find this essential oil listed as simply "geranium." Either botanical name is accurate. The fresh, roselike, "green" scent with uplifting and balancing qualities is derived from leaves, stalks, and flowers. When inhaled, it helps relieve stress, fatigue, and anxiety. Use this stimulating, slightly astringent oil to help alleviate water retention in the legs resulting from poor circulation. It makes a good addition to anticellulite massage oil blends and facial elixirs formulated for mature, combination, and environmentally damaged skin, but because it helps to balance sebum production, it can be used for all skin types.

Ginger (*Zingiber officinalis*)

PARTS USED: **Essential oil (CO_2 extract)**

COSMETIC PROPERTIES AND USES: The spicy, warming, soft aroma of this oil is great for massage oil blends to ease muscle aches and pains. The relaxing and grounding scent also makes it a helpful addition to sleep-enhancing balms.

CONTRAINDICATIONS: Avoid if pregnant or epileptic. May be a potential skin irritant.

Glycerin, Vegetable

COSMETIC PROPERTIES AND USES: Derived from vegetable fats, this is clear, slippery, moisturizing, and sweet-tasting and acts as a humectant (it draws moisture from the air to the skin). It's a good addition to lotions and creams specifically formulated to rehydrate skin. Water-soluble glycerin is much lighter than a base oil. Use it as a sweet flavoring agent in personal lubricants and edible, flavored body balms.

Grapefruit *(Citrus paradisii)*

PARTS USED: Essential oil

COSMETIC PROPERTIES AND USES: The sparkling, sweet-tart, stimulating aroma helps balance moods and lift spirits. Add it to massage oil blends to alleviate water retention and cellulite. In facial elixirs it is a specific for congested, acneic, and combination skin. This oil has a calming effect on the psyche. Use it in sleep-enhancing balms.

CONTRAINDICATIONS: Avoid if pregnant or epileptic. May be photosensitizing and a potential skin irritant.

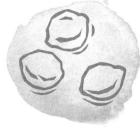

Hazelnut Oil *(Corylus americana)*

COSMETIC PROPERTIES AND USES: This highly penetrative base oil derived from the hazelnut is virtually identical in quality, color, and recommended usages to apricot kernel oil (page 59).

POSSIBLE SUBSTITUTES: Apricot kernel, almond, or soybean oil

Helichrysum *(Helichrysum italicum var. serotinum)*

PARTS USED: Essential oil

COSMETIC PROPERTIES AND USES: Also known as Everlasting or Immortelle, this essential oil is steam-distilled from flowers. Highly aromatic, with warm, herbal undertones, it's a very potent anti-inflammatory and antirheumatic. It's indicated for use in healing bruises, sprains, open wounds and cuts, acne, eczema, and psoriasis. When blended with rose hip seed base oil, it helps reduce the appearance of scar tissue and stretch marks. It also stimulates new cell formation.

Honey, Raw

COSMETIC PROPERTIES AND USES: Sweet, sticky honey acts as a humectant (see Glycerin, Vegetable, page 71). Use it in hydrating, soothing masks for all skin types or to sweeten lip balms and edible body balms.

Hops *(Humulus lupulus)*

PARTS USED: Conelike fruit or strobilae

COSMETIC PROPERTIES AND USES: This bitter herb commonly used in the beer-brewing industry is recommended medicinally for its calming effect on the nervous system and to help overcome insomnia. Inhaling its aroma or taking it in tincture form helps to ease tension and anxiety. Combine hops with more fragrant sedating herbs such as rose petals, lavender buds, sweet marjoram, and lemon balm in making herbal sleep pillows.

Hydrosols, Aromatic (a.k.a. Flower Waters)

COSMETIC PROPERTIES AND USES: Aromatic hydrosols are a natural by-product of the essential oil distillation process. These fragrant waters are saturated with compounds present in specific plants and are gentle enough to use when an essential oil would be too irritating to a particular skin type or condition. Hydrosols are packaged in spray bottles and can be used as air fresheners and facial spritzers or toners to rehydrate dry skin or to cool a hot flash. Spray them in your surroundings to energize or relax your mind, or add to lotion and cream recipes.

CHAMOMILE *(Anthemis nobilis* or *Matricaria chamomilla)*
This soothing and balancing hydrosol is good for all skin types, especially sensitive, irritated, environmentally damaged, or mature skin. It acts as a gentle, calming agent for skin and psyche with a floral, apple-like, relaxing fragrance.

GERANIUM, ROSE *(Pelargonium graveolens)*
The clean, roselike aroma of this hydrosol lifts the spirits. Slightly astringent, it balances all skin types, especially mature, combination, and environmentally damaged skin. Used as a facial spritzer, it's cooling for hot flashes. It also eliminates stale odors.

LAVENDER *(Lavandula angustifolia)*
This classic hydrosol has a clean, fresh fragrance that's similar to that of lavender buds. Its gentle astringent, antiseptic, calming, and healing qualities bring relief to skin irritations and sunburn, but it's good for all skin types.

LEMON BALM *(Melissa officinalis)*

The tart, citruslike aroma of this hydrosol uplifts a "down" mood and calms mental stress. Highly anti-inflammatory, it's beneficial and cooling when used on "angry," red, acneic skin; cold sores; herpes outbreaks; eczema; psoriasis; and general dermatitis. It can be used on all skin types, especially those in need of soothing.

NEROLI OR ORANGE BLOSSOM *(Citrus aurantium)*

The delicate fragrance is reminiscent of orange blossoms and jasmine with a hint of cool "green." One of my favorites, it acts as a mild, refreshing astringent and assists in sebum regulation. It's beneficial to acneic, irritated, oily, sensitive, environmentally damaged, or mature skin.

ROSE OTTO *(Rosa damascena)*

This has a subtle, warm, floral aroma and acts as a light astringent for all skin types, calming and soothing redness. It also relaxes the mind, eases anxiety, and serves as a mood-setting room spray.

ROSEMARY *(Rosmarinus officinalis)*

With its refreshing, cooling, herbaceous fragrance, this hydrosol acts as a stimulating, mild astringent for oily and normal skin and improves sluggish circulation. Keep a bottle in the office for an afternoon aromatic pick-me-up. Spray the surrounding air, your hair, wrists, face, and neck — it will help to lift mental fog and energize your thought processes.

Jojoba Oil *(Simmondsia chinensis)*

COSMETIC PROPERTIES AND USES: A medium-textured base oil (technically a liquid wax ester) derived from pressed plant seeds or beans and chemically similar to our own moisturizing sebum, jojoba penetrates well, leaving no oily residue. It's one of my favorite base oils for perfume, facial elixirs, and bath and massage oil blends because it does not turn rancid and requires no refrigeration. It's also an excellent conditioner for hair, scalp, skin, and nails and is an all-purpose skin lubricant.

POSSIBLE SUBSTITUTES: Sunflower seed oil, but it does not have the same shelf life as jojoba and doesn't penetrate as well.

Juniper Berry (*Juniperus communis*)

PARTS USED: Essential oil, berries

COSMETIC PROPERTIES AND USES: The refreshing, woody-sweet fragrance uplifts and stimulates to improve productivity and alertness. Use the berries in herbal bath blends to relieve sore muscles. The essential oil can be used in balms to comfort the pain of arthritis and muscle strain as well as in facial elixirs to balance oily skin and acne. Juniper essential oil has a strong diuretic action, which makes it a good addition to anticellulite bath and massage oil blends.

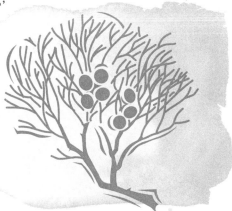

POSSIBLE SUBSTITUTES: Eucalyptus (*E. radiata*) or peppermint essential oils for easing sore muscles, but these don't have the same diuretic action as juniper. Rose geranium essential oil can be substituted for Juniper in an anticellulite recipe.

CONTRAINDICATIONS: Avoid essential oil if pregnant or epileptic or if you have kidney problems. May also be a potential skin irritant.

Lady's Mantle (*Alchemilla vulgaris*)

PARTS USED: Leaves

COSMETIC PROPERTIES AND USES: Healing and soothing, as an infusion or tea it makes a light astringent for normal-to-dry or sensitive skin. It's particularly good for weeping acne when a stronger astringent might further sting and irritate already aggravated skin.

POSSIBLE SUBSTITUTES: Calendula blossoms or elder flowers

Lanolin, Anhydrous

COSMETIC PROPERTIES AND USES: Occasionally called wool fat or wool wax, lanolin is derived from the sebaceous glands of sheep and is secreted into their wool as a protective agent against cold and dampness. Because it's similar to the natural oil in human skin, it makes a fantastic moisturizer. A thick, animal wax with a wool-like aroma, it helps prevent skin dehydration. In moisturizers, lanolin is a water-absorbing emulsifier that improves the emollient effect of creams and lotions and aids in the stabilization of these oil and water blends.

CONTRAINDICATIONS: May possibly cause contact allergic skin rashes in very sensitive skin, though I have not seen this in my practice. Be sure to purchase only pure or anhydrous lanolin versus hydrolyzed lanolin, which is more readily available and is practically odorless, but is often heavily processed and laden with chemicals.

Lavender *(Lavandula angustifolia)*

PARTS USED: Flower buds, essential oil

COSMETIC PROPERTIES AND USES: The mature buds can be made into an infusion or tea for use as a soothing face wash or toner for all skin types, especially irritated and acneic skin. Combine dried, ground flowers with powdered oatmeal and roses and use as a calming face cleanser and mask for even the most sensitive skin.

Lavender essential oil is one of the most gentle, universally useful essential oils, with an old-fashioned, soft, floral and herbal scent. It can be used neat, or undiluted, on the skin. Its aroma is known for its relaxing, calming effect on the central nervous system. About five minutes before giving live radio interviews, or skin care demonstrations, I take several deep inhalations of lavender essential oil directly from the bottle to calm my nervous jitters. Sedative, antispasmodic, and antiseptic, this essential oil is a must for all first-aid kits. It can be used to relieve sunburns, insect bites, cuts, blemishes, headaches, muscular aches, painful sinuses, colds, flu, and menstrual cramps and can induce sleep in the most chronic insomniac.

Lemon (*Citrus limonum*)

PARTS USED: Juice, essential oil, rind

COSMETIC PROPERTIES AND USES: The clean, light, citrus aroma has uplifting, invigorating properties. The diluted juice acts as a moderate-to-strong astringent and disinfectant and as mild bleach, benefiting unbalanced, blotchy, oily, and acneic skin and helping to restore natural skin pH. Use the dried, powdered rind in face and body scrubs and the essential oil — sparingly — in face cleansers and body lotions.

POSSIBLE SUBSTITUTES: Tangerine juice for its astringent property, and tangerine essential oil primarily for its fragrance. Dried, powdered orange rind can be substituted for lemon rind.

CONTRAINDICATIONS: Avoid essential oil if pregnant or epileptic. May be photosensitizing and a potential skin irritant.

Lemon Balm (*Melissa officinalis*)

PARTS USED: Leaves, essential oil

COSMETIC PROPERTIES AND USES: Also known as Melissa, true lemon balm essential oil, with its heady, tart, "green" aroma, acts as a sedative, antidepressant, and potent antiviral and is rare and very expensive but worth the price if you can manage to purchase a tiny bottle. Lemon balm essential oil is primarily used in natural perfumes and personal care recipes for its aromatic and skin-soothing qualities. It blends well with other floral and citrus oils and vanilla. Use the fresh or dried leaves in mild astringents for normal and dry skin, but because it is so gentle, it can be enjoyed by all skin types. The dried leaves also make a good addition to sleep-enhancing pillows.

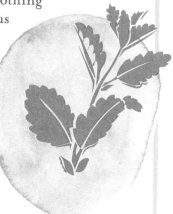

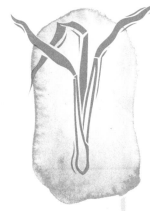

Lemongrass (*Cymbopogon citratus*)

PARTS USED: Leaves, essential oil

COSMETIC PROPERTIES AND USES: Lemongrass, with its astringent, anti-viral, and antibacterial qualities, has a stimulating, pungent, earthy, lemony scent. Both the herbal infusion or tea and essential oil are used in creams, lotions, and skin cleansers formulated for normal and oily skin. Lemongrass essential oil, derived from the grasslike leaves, acts as a natural insect repellent and is frequently combined with citronella and catnip essential oils in natural bug-deterrent sprays. It also makes a fantastic room deodorizer, especially around cat litter boxes.

CONTRAINDICATIONS: Avoid essential oil if pregnant or epileptic. May be a potential skin irritant.

Macadamia Nut Oil (*Macadamia integrifolia*)

COSMETIC PROPERTIES AND USES: This light- to medium-textured, penetrating base oil is high in monounsaturated fatty acids. Like jojoba and sunflower seed oils, it closely resembles the chemical makeup of sebum. Use it in facial elixirs for mature or environmentally damaged skin and skin that's irritated, sunburned, or windburned. It's often used in blends to help soften scar tissue.

Marjoram, Sweet (*Origanum majorana*)

PARTS USED: Leaves, essential oil

COSMETIC PROPERTIES AND USES: This tasty culinary plant is also helpful at relieving pent-up anxiety, tension, and insomnia. The dried leaves can be used in making dream pillows to help induce relaxation and calmness. The essential oil, derived from leaves and flowers, has a woody, herbal, cool aroma that can be used for its tranquilizing properties in making sleep-enhancing balms. It also acts as a respiratory disinfectant.

CONTRAINDICATIONS: Avoid use of essential oil if pregnant or epileptic.

Marsh Mallow (*Althaea officinalis*)

PARTS USED: Root

COSMETIC PROPERTIES AND USES: The Greek word *althaea* means "to heal." Marsh mallow root contains a soothing mucilage that, when steeped in simmering water, produces a slippery, healing "goo" that is quite beneficial for weather-beaten, chapped, or sun-damaged skin. It's good for all skin types, but especially those needing added moisture and comfort for irritated tissues. (See Comfrey, on page 68, for similar properties.)

POSSIBLE SUBSTITUTES: Comfrey root

Milk, Whole Dried

COSMETIC PROPERTIES AND USES: Whole milk is high in skin-softening lipids (fats) and mild, exfoliating lactic acid. It makes a pampering bath additive and skin cleanser for normal, dry, and sensitive skin.

POSSIBLE SUBSTITUTES: Nonfat dried milk mixed with a few drops of almond, soybean, jojoba, extra-virgin olive, or macadamia nut oil to compensate for its lack of natural fat.

Myrrh (*Commiphora myrrha*)

PARTS USED: Tincture of myrrh, myrrh powder, essential oil

COSMETIC PROPERTIES AND USES: Tincture of myrrh, an alcohol extract of the tree resin or gum, has a rich, heavy aroma and acts as an antiseptic, astringent, and disinfectant. It's good for sores in the mouth and throat, sore teeth, irritated or infected gums, and bad breath, and can also be applied directly to fresh cuts, scrapes, and bug bites to prevent infection and speed healing. It acts as a natural cosmetic preservative as well. Powdered myrrh is used in body powders as a natural deodorizer, and the essential oil is used in mouthwashes, facial creams, and lotions for its astringent and anti-inflammatory properties.

CONTRAINDICATIONS: Avoid essential oil if pregnant or epileptic.

Myrtle, Green (*Myrtus communis*)

PARTS USED: Essential oil

COSMETIC PROPERTIES AND USES: Derived from leaves and flowers, the fragrance is similar to fresh, camphorous eucalyptus, but is softer and more delicate. Its vapors help open sinuses and decongest lungs. It's used on oily, combination, or acneic skin due to its antiseptic and astringent actions. The aroma is said to quell anger, calm emotional upset, and lift a "down" mood.

CONTRAINDICATIONS: Avoid essential oil if pregnant or epileptic.

Neem (*Azadirachta indica*)

PARTS USED: Base oil, leaves

COSMETIC PROPERTIES AND USES: A rich, thick, golden-brown base oil with a strong nutty aroma, neem oil is generally diluted with sesame, jojoba, or extra-virgin olive oils to improve pourability. Derived from pressed neem tree nuts, it has antiseptic, antiviral, antifungal, insecticidal, and antibacterial properties. It solidifies at a cool room temperature. Neem is excellent for use in antidandruff treatments, anti-acne elixirs, and antifungal remedies for feet and nails. It has a low SPF and can be blended with sesame and jojoba base oils for use in natural sunscreen recipes. It can also be used as an additive in natural insect repellents. Use the dried leaves in soap-free herbal hair wash formulas to help relieve scalp irritations and itching.

Neroli (*Citrus aurantium*)

PARTS USED: Essential oil

COSMETIC PROPERTIES AND USES: This is one of my favorite essential oils. Gentle to the skin and soothing to the psyche, it has a rich, erotic, delicate, orange-blossom aroma. It can be used on all skin types but is especially beneficial to mature and environmentally damaged skin. Use it in facial elixirs to promote cell regeneration and improve elasticity. Many consider this oil to be an aphrodisiac, making it a good addition to massage oil recipes. It blends well with other floral, citrus, and woody essential oils.

Nettle *(Urtica dioica)*

PARTS USED: **Leaves**

COSMETIC PROPERTIES AND USES: A strong infusion or tea can be used as a mineral-rich astringent for oily-to-normal, combination, or acneic skin. Nettle is a classic ingredient in herbal shampoos, hair rinses, and hair growth formulas for dark hair. It stimulates circulation.

POSSIBLE SUBSTITUTES: Rosemary leaves

Nonpetroleum Jelly

COSMETIC PROPERTIES AND USES: This is a commercially available alternative to petroleum jelly, with a similar thick, emollient consistency. Made from a combination of vegetable oils, this jelly can be used in a pinch to heal and soothe chapped lips, dermatitis, dry cuticles, dry heels, elbows, and knees.

Oatmeal *(Avena sativa)*

PARTS USED: Old-fashioned oatmeal, ground into a fine, flourlike meal

COSMETIC PROPERTIES AND USES: Soothing to all types of skin irritations and sensitivities, oatmeal makes a gentle abrasive base for face and body scrubs, powdered cleansers, masks, and bath bags. Colloidal oatmeal, available in better drug stores, is ground extremely fine, can be poured directly into the bathtub, and is recommended for relieving the itch caused by poison ivy; poison oak; and rashy, dry, sensitive skin.

Olive Oil, Extra-Virgin *(Olea europaea)*

COSMETIC PROPERTIES AND USES: This green, rich, moderately heavy base oil with a strong olive aroma is derived from the first pressing of ripe olives and is high in beneficial vitamins and minerals. It can be blended with a lighter-textured, odorless base oil in body care products. It's wonderful as a makeup remover and skin softener, though completely masking its fragrance can be difficult. When color and fragrance aren't a concern, however, such as in medicinal salves, many herbalists use it exclusively. Used alone, it makes an excellent conditioning oil for dry hair, nails, and feet.

POSSIBLE SUBSTITUTES: Avocado or jojoba base oils

Orange, Sweet (*Citrus sinensis*)

PARTS USED: Dried rind or peel, essential oil

COSMETIC PROPERTIES AND USES: The ground, dried peel is used in aromatic bath bags and body scrubs. The sweet, fruity essential oil is used in creams and lotions for oily-to-normal and combination skin and in anticellulite formulas. The aroma has a sedative, calming effect and helps relieve anxiety. The essential oil can be used as a flavoring agent in lip balms, edible body balms, and children's formulas.

POSSIBLE SUBSTITUTES: Tangerine essential oil for its astringent and fragrant properties.

CONTRAINDICATIONS: Avoid if pregnant or epileptic. May be photosensitizing and a potential skin irritant.

Papaya (*Carica papaya*)

PARTS USED: Fresh, raw mashed pulp, unpasteurized juice

COSMETIC PROPERTIES AND USES: Papaya contains *papain,* a protein-digesting enzyme which helps dissolve the dead outer layer of skin, revealing the new layer underneath. Use papaya when making masks for almost any skin type, but particularly for skin that's in need of deep cleansing, brightening, and balancing of uneven coloration. It really helps rid skin of a blotchy appearance.

CONTRAINDICATIONS: Avoid use on irritated, sensitive, sunburned, or windburned skin.

Parsley (*Petroselinum sativum*)

PARTS USED: Leaves

COSMETIC PROPERTIES AND USES: A parsley infusion is gently astringent, soothing, and healing for those who suffer from weeping acne, eczema, psoriasis, or any irritable dermatitis. It also makes a hair rinse to combat dandruff and flaky scalp. Chew the leaves for a classic breath freshener.

Peach (*Prunus persica*)

PARTS USED: Fresh, mashed pulp, unpasteurized juice

COSMETIC PROPERTIES AND USES: Nourishing, moisturizing, and toning for all skin types, peach also has a yummy fruity fragrance. Mix the pulp or juice with heavy cream for a super-emollient, dry-skin-pampering mask.

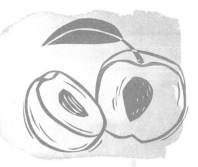

Peppermint (*Mentha piperita*)

PARTS USED: Leaves, essential oil

COSMETIC PROPERTIES AND USES: Peppermint is a true multipurpose herb. An infusion of the leaves — cooling, deodorizing, stimulating, astringent, and antiseptic — is good for oily-to-normal, combination, and acneic skin. Peppermint infusion can be made into a deodorizing body splash and foot bath, a breath-freshening gargle, and a mouthwash. The essential oil is commonly used in natural dentifrice recipes and cooling body lotions and creams. When it's inhaled, it energizes and awakens the mind. It also makes a terrific room freshener.

POSSIBLE SUBSTITUTES: Spearmint leaves and essential oil, though they're not as strong in fragrance or action.

CONTRAINDICATIONS: Avoid if pregnant or epileptic.

Pineapple (*Ananas comosus*)

PARTS USED: Fresh, raw juice strained from the mashed pulp

COSMETIC PROPERTIES AND USES: Containing *bromelain*, a protein-digesting enzyme, pineapple dissolves dead surface skin cells, resulting in softer, smoother skin. It works like papaya (see page 82). Use the astringent juice in facial masks for all skin types, particularly those in need of brightening, gentle bleaching, and deep cleansing.

CONTRAINDICATIONS: Avoid use on sensitive, sunburned, windburned, or irritated skin.

Raspberry, Red (*Rubus idaeus*)

PARTS USED: Leaves; freshly pressed, strained fruit juice

COSMETIC PROPERTIES AND USES: The infused leaves are gently astringent and have similar properties as blackberry and strawberry leaves. Good for oily-to-normal and combination skin, the fresh juice contains lactic acid (like milk or yogurt) and, when applied to the skin, acts as a nonabrasive exfoliant, removing dead-skin buildup.

POSSIBLE SUBSTITUTES: Strawberry or blackberry leaves or fresh strawberry juice

CONTRAINDICATIONS: Avoid use of fresh juice if skin is sensitive, irritated, sunburned, or windburned.

Ravensara (*Ravensara aromatica*)

PARTS USED: Essential oil

COSMETIC PROPERTIES AND USES: Derived from plant leaves, this oil has a camphorous, sinus-stimulating aroma akin to traditional eucalyptus but lighter and fresher. It's one of my favorite inhalants for clearing a stuffy head, raising overall energy, and lifting mental fog, though some find it relaxing instead of energizing. An effective antiviral, this oil can be used in sinus balms and chest rubs. You can also add it to facial elixirs to help treat herpes, cold sores, and cold and flu symptoms.

POSSIBLE SUBSTITUTES: *Eucalyptus radiata*

CONTRAINDICATIONS: Avoid if pregnant or epileptic.

Rose Otto (*Rosa damascena*)

PARTS USED: Petals, essential oil

COSMETIC PROPERTIES AND USES: Rose essential oil is very expensive yet exquisite, with a deep, complex, true-rose aroma. Valued for use as a skin cell regenerator, mild astringent, mood elevator, and aphrodisiac, use this oil in formulas for all skin types, especially mature and environmentally damaged skin. It also adds a wonderful scent in body powders and body balms for infants and young girls. The dried powdered petals (*Rosa gallica* or *centifolia* species) are generally dark pink or deep red in color and are used in powdered face cleanser recipes. The dried whole petals are used in facial steams.

Rose Hip Seed Oil (*Rosa rubiginosa*)

COSMETIC PROPERTIES AND USES: Available commercially as Rosa Mosqueta oil, this is a medium to heavy, pale, orange-red base oil derived from the seeds of the Andean rose hip. When very fresh, it has a light, tart aroma. High in essential fatty acids, it's ideal for mature, environmentally damaged, prematurely aged, and devitalized skin. Use this oil combined with calophyllum (see page 63) in facial elixirs and creams specifically to rejuvenate, soften, and heal skin damaged by scars, stretch marks, and extreme weather exposure.

CONTRAINDICATIONS: Avoid use on oily, acneic, or combination skin; this oil may further exacerbate these conditions.

Rosemary (*Rosmarinus officinalis*)

PARTS USED: Leaves, essential oil (chemotype *verbenon*)

COSMETIC PROPERTIES AND USES: The *verbenon* chemotype (as opposed to the chemotypes *camphor* and *cineol*) is the preferred variety for skin care, with its crisp, lemony aroma and sedative effects. Use it in bath and massage oils and facial elixirs for toning oily-to-normal and combination skin and for its cell regenerating and antiseptic properties. It also helps open sinuses, heal wounds, and stimulate new hair growth. It blends very well with lavender, basil, and lemon essential oils as a hair and scalp conditioner and growth enhancer. An infusion of the leaves can be used as a darkening hair rinse and also cleanses and refreshes an oily scalp and relieves dandruff.

CONTRAINDICATIONS: Avoid use of the essential oil if pregnant or epileptic.

Sage (*Salvia officinalis*)

PARTS USED: Leaves

COSMETIC PROPERTIES AND USES: This multipurpose plant has a classic, pungent, herbal, spicy, "Thanksgiving" scent. The infusion or tea is used as an astringent and antiseptic for oily, combination, acneic, and normal skin; a rinse to darken hair; a disinfectant for minor cuts, abrasions, and insect bites; a foot deodorizer; and a sore-throat gargle.

POSSIBLE SUBSTITUTES: Strong, rosemary leaf infusion

Sea Salt, Fine Ground

COSMETIC PROPERTIES AND USES: This salt is healing and drying to open sores and pimples. (You may have noticed how quickly blemishes or minor cuts heal after swimming in the ocean.) Use sea salt in body and foot scrub recipes as an abrasive exfoliant to slough away rough skin. You can also combine sea salt with baking soda to use as a natural dentifrice, or combine the two and add essential oils and dried herbs for use as scented, pampering bath salts.

CONTRAINDICATIONS: Do not use if skin is dry, sensitive, or irritated in any way. Also, sea salt is much too abrasive for the face area; use only on the body.

Sesame Seed Oil (*Sesamum indicum*)

COSMETIC PROPERTIES AND USES: Derived from pressed sesame seeds, this clear, sometimes pale yellow, antioxidant base oil has a distinct aroma and is rich in vitamins A and E and protein. It's stable, with a long shelf life, though I still prefer to refrigerate it and use it within one year. It has a low natural SPF and thus can be used in natural sunscreen recipes. It also makes a penetrating, relaxing body and massage oil and is recommended for use on normal-to-dry skin. *Note:* Do not use the toasted variety of sesame oil in your skin care recipes to avoid an aroma that's reminiscent of "essence of Asian stir-fry"!

POSSIBLE SUBSTITUTES: Sunflower seed oil

Shampoo Base: Natural, Plain, and Unscented

COSMETIC PROPERTIES AND USES: When making natural shampoos, bubble baths, face cleansers, and body washes, some people prefer to use a natural shampoo base instead of liquid castile soap (which, especially when used on curly, fine, thin, dry, and chemically-treated hair, can leave a gummy soap residue despite sufficient rinsing and can contribute to tangles, snarls, and a dull appearance). Also, if skin is already dry or dehydrated, castile soap can dry it further. A natural shampoo base using plant-derived decyl polyglucose or olefin sulphonate as the foaming and cleansing agents is a superior, nonstripping base for homemade formulas.

Look for shampoo base either online from natural cosmetic ingredient suppliers, in better health food stores, or from some herb catalogs. If you can't find a product labeled "base," then a natural baby shampoo could work in a pinch.

CONTRAINDICATIONS: Natural shampoo base is generally gentle enough for all hair types, but, like all soaps, it shouldn't be used as a cleanser for skin that tends to be dry or irritated.

Shea Butter *(Butyrospermum parkii)*

COSMETIC PROPERTIES AND USES: Derived from the pressed nuts of the karite tree, in its unrefined form shea butter is a cream-colored, soft substance with a strong fragrance that's difficult to mask. If the scent displeases you, then purchase the white, refined butter. It will be firmer, but will have the same properties. (I actually prefer this product in the refined form.) Shea butter is a highly emollient, skin-softening additive in lotions, creams, body balms, and nail care and after-sun care recipes. It can even be used alone if desired.

Soybean Oil *(Soyas hispida)*

COSMETIC PROPERTIES AND USES: A light-textured, pale-golden base oil that is easily absorbed, this makes a terrific massage oil and facial elixir base for all skin types. I use it as the primary base oil for body balms and some creams; it lends velvety texture when combined with beeswax, cocoa butter, and shea butter. Soybean oil has natural insect-repellent properties and thus is frequently used as the base oil in chemical-free bug repellents. *Note:* Purchase only organic soybean oil. The soybean oil in the grocery store is generally labeled "vegetable oil" and is highly refined at high temperatures and chock-full of chemical residue.

POSSIBLE SUBSTITUTES: Sunflower seed, hazelnut, or almond oil, though they don't provide quite the same texture to balms and creams as does soybean oil.

Strawberry (*Fragaria vesca*)

PARTS USED: Leaves, mashed fruit pulp, and juice

COSMETIC PROPERTIES AND USES: An infusion or tea of the leaves makes a gentle astringent or body splash for oily-to-normal or combination skin. Use the berry pulp to freshen breath and whiten teeth. Use the fresh-pressed juice in masks for oily-to-normal or combination skin or apply it directly onto pimples as a healing, drying aid. It contains a gentle, exfoliating acid that helps to rid skin of dead-cell buildup.

POSSIBLE SUBSTITUTES: Blackberry or raspberry leaves. There is no substitute for the fruit.

Sugar, White or Brown, Fine Granulated

COSMETIC PROPERTIES AND USES: Sugar can be used as an abrasive exfoliant just like sea salt in body and foot scrub recipes, but because it doesn't dry or sting the skin, many prefer it to sea salt. Sugar contains natural glycolic acids, meaning it also exfoliates on a chemical level, rather than by abrasion alone.

CONTRAINDICATIONS: Avoid use on abraded, irritated, sunburned, windburned, or sensitive skin. Sugar is too abrasive to be used on the face; use only on the body.

Sunflower Seed Meal (*Helianthus annus*)

PARTS USED: Raw seeds ground into a medium-fine meal

COSMETIC PROPERTIES AND USES: Rich in essential fatty acids, emollients, and nutrients, sunflower seed meal makes a gentle, moisturizing face and body scrub and facial mask base for normal-to-dry skin. Because of its high fat content and the softness of its granules, it can be used to exfoliate even sensitive and acneic skin, but always use a gentle touch.

POSSIBLE SUBSTITUTES: Almond meal, if very finely ground

CONTRAINDICATIONS: Do not use on irritated, sunburned, or windburned skin.

Sunflower Seed Oil (*Helianthus annus*)

COSMETIC PROPERTIES AND USES: This is a light- to medium-textured base oil high in essential fatty acids; antioxidant vitamins A, D, and E; and lecithin derived from pressed seeds. Deeply nourishing and moisturizing for all skin types except oily, it's similar to human sebum. Use this all-purpose inexpensive oil in all lotions, creams, bath and massage oil blends, body balms, and hair conditioning oil recipes.

POSSIBLE SUBSTITUTES: Almond, soybean, or macadamia oil

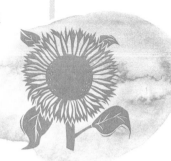

Tangerine (*Citrus reticulata*)

PARTS USED: Essential oil

COSMETIC PROPERTIES AND USES: Derived from the pressed peel, this has a tart, sweet, uplifting, soothing aroma. It's slightly astringent and, because of its flavor and aromatic properties, can be used primarily as a substitute for sweet orange essential oil in lip balms, body lotions, creams, and edible body balms.

POSSIBLE SUBSTITUTES: Sweet orange essential oil

CONTRAINDICATIONS: Avoid if pregnant or epileptic. May be photosensitizing and a potential skin irritant.

Tea Tree (*Melaleuca alternifolia*)

PARTS USED: Essential oil

COSMETIC PROPERTIES AND USES: A very safe essential oil with a strong, camphorous, balsamic, medicinal odor derived from the plant leaves, this is a potent antibacterial, antifungal, and antiviral. It makes an excellent addition to the home medicine chest. It helps heal acne, open wounds, cuts, infections, rashes, and dermatitis and works well in cleansers, astringents, facial elixirs, and masks for acneic and blemish-prone skin. It can be used neat (undiluted) as a spot treatment for pimples.

POSSIBLE SUBSTITUTES: Lavender essential oil, though it's not as powerful in medicinal properties.

Thyme (Thymus vulgaris)

PARTS USED: **Essential oil (chemotype** *linalol*)**, leaves**

COSMETIC PROPERTIES AND USES: Derived from the plant leaves, this special chemotype of thyme essential oil is skin-friendly and gentle, unlike red thyme (*Thymus vulgaris* chemotype *thymol*), which is hot and irritating. It has a sweet, "green," lightly medicinal aroma and is an effective antiseptic and antibacterial agent. It's healing for weeping acne and rashes resulting from poison oak, poison ivy, and sumac or general contact dermatitis. Use it in cleansers, astringents, lotions, facial elixirs, and masks for acneic and blemish-prone skin and in sinus and cold- and flu-preventive balms, salves, and elixirs. An infusion of thyme leaves produces an astringent liquid for an oily, combination, or normal complexion or as a cleansing wound wash. Powdered thyme is a good antibacterial and deodorizing agent in body and foot powders.

POSSIBLE SUBSTITUTES: Tea tree essential oil may be substituted for thyme essential oil, though it has a much more penetrating, medicinal odor.

CONTRAINDICATIONS: Avoid use of essential oil if you are pregnant or epileptic or have high blood pressure. May be a potential skin irritant for sensitive skin.

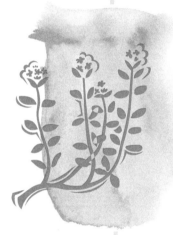

Vanilla (Vanilla planifolia)

PARTS USED: **Essential oil, whole vanilla beans**

COSMETIC PROPERTIES AND USES: This sweet, rich, familiar fragrance is derived from the vanilla bean. It balances mood and reduces stress, is a calming aphrodisiac, and softens all fragrance blends. The essential oil can be used in relaxing massage oil blends; fragrant creams; and as a flavoring and scent in edible body balms, lip balms, and personal lubricants. You can slice open and chop vanilla beans for use in an infused base oil for bath and massage oil recipes. To make a highly aromatic edible oil, infuse vanilla beans in liquefied, organic, unrefined coconut oil. (The best time to make this base oil is during warm weather, above 76°F, so that the coconut oil doesn't harden.) *Note:* If you are a fan of all things vanilla, look for vanilla bean paste, a vanilla flavoring that is thick with vanilla bean seeds and sweetened with sugar, and keep a bottle on hand to add to edible body balms.

Vitamin E Oil *(D–Alpha Tocopherol or Mixed Tocopherols)*

PARTS USED: Capsule form, measured in international units (IU)

COSMETIC PROPERTIES AND USES: This antioxidant oil acts as a preservative when added to other base oils, lotions, and creams by preventing rancidity of fatty ingredients. When topically applied, it aids in prevention of scar tissue resulting from burns, weight gain, pregnancy, cuts, wounds, and surgery.

CONTRAINDICATIONS: Because it may irritate eyes and sensitive skin, use this heavy-textured oil on the body alone, not on the face area.

Vodka

COSMETIC PROPERTIES AND USES: Commonly derived from the fermentation of potatoes or grain, this fragrance-free alcoholic product can be used as an extractive solvent in herbal, alcohol-based toners for oily, normal, and combination skin; herbal perfumes; and men's aftershave formulas. Always purchase vodka that's 80 or 100 proof.

CONTRAINDICATIONS: Avoid applying to dry, irritated, sensitive, sunburned, windburned, or abraded skin.

Walnut, Black (*Juglans nigra*)

PARTS USED: **Nut hulls**

COSMETIC PROPERTIES AND USES: A walnut infusion is very astringent. When hulls are simmered in water, they produce a dark brown liquid that can be used as a rinse to brighten or add a hint of red to black or brunette hair or darken light-colored hair. Use only if you have oily-to-normal scalp and hair. *Note:* A walnut-hull infusion will *not* radically darken hair or penetrate the hair's cuticle as a chemical dye does, though it will temporarily stain blond, reddish-blond, or light brown hair a darker shade. This color will fade after a few shampoos unless you are a "chemical blond," in which case the infusion may react unpleasantly with the unnatural color of your hair. Be aware of this potential chemical reaction.

CONTRAINDICATIONS: Avoid use on a dry scalp or dry, damaged hair; it may cause further dehydration and dryness. A walnut-hull infusion will stain hands, nails, and light-colored towels a light shade of brown. Take the proper precautions when using this dark liquid.

Water, Distilled

COSMETIC PROPERTIES AND USES: When making personal care products that call for water or when making herbal infusions or tea, toners, astringents, or splashes, always use distilled water. This type of water is void of bacteria and will not introduce contaminants into your products. Tap water should not be used (unless it is the only water source) because it contains chemicals and waterborne bacteria. If you must use tap water, boil it first. Purified, filtered, or bottled water can be used if distilled water is unavailable.

Wheat Germ *(Triticum aestivum)*

PARTS USED: Raw, fresh wheat germ

COSMETIC PROPERTIES AND USES: Wheat germ is the heart of the wheat kernel. Due to its high fat content, it becomes rancid quickly if stored at room temperature. Fresh, raw wheat germ usually can be found in the refrigerator or freezer section of your local health food store. If you don't find it in either place, leave it on the shelf! It's rich in protein, essential fatty acids, vitamins B and E, and soluble dietary fiber. Use in nourishing, softening facial masks for normal-to-very dry, environmentally damaged, and mature skin. It's especially good for sensitive, irritated, sunburned, and windburned complexions.

Witch Hazel *(Hamamelis virginiana)*

PARTS USED: Bark or commercially prepared liquid

COSMETIC PROPERTIES AND USES: For convenience, the commercially prepared liquid is used most often. It consists primarily of water with added witch hazel alcohol extract and acts as a gentle, nearly unscented astringent for oily-to-normal and combination skin.

CONTRAINDICATIONS: Avoid use on dry, sensitive, sunburned, or windburned skin.

Yarrow *(Achillea millefolium)*

PARTS USED: Leaves, flowers

COSMETIC PROPERTIES AND USES: Yarrow is also known as milfoil or soldier's wound wort because it was valued on the battlefield for closing wounds and arresting bleeding due to its strong astringent and styptic properties. The herbal infusion makes a potent astringent for oily, acneic, combination, and normal skin. It also makes a healing wash for all kinds of precleansed wounds and sores.

CONTRAINDICATIONS: Avoid use on dry or dehydrated skin. Extended use may make skin photosensitive.

Ylang Ylang (*Cananga odorata*)

PARTS USED: **Essential oil**

COSMETIC PROPERTIES AND USES: This sweet, slightly sticky, spicy and floral essential oil rivals rose and jasmine oils as one of the most exotic aromas on earth. The scent relaxes muscles as well as the central nervous system, balances mood, calms the mind, and acts as an antidepressant. The oil also regulates sebum production for all skin types. Use it in body and massage oil recipes and in floral perfumes; body balms; creams; and sleep-enhancing balms. It blends well with citrus, spice, floral, and cedar essential oils. When anxious, inhale ylang ylang oil directly from the bottle or apply it to pulse points.

Yogurt, Plain

PARTS USED: Comes in sheep, cow, or goat varieties that are full-fat, low-fat, or nonfat. No additives, thickeners, or stabilizers, please.

COSMETIC PROPERTIES AND USES: Try to purchase raw yogurt if available, but pasteurized will work fine. Acting as a mild, nonabrasive, bleaching exfoliant, it contains natural lactic acid, which helps dissolve surface dead-skin cells, leaving behind soft, evenly toned skin. It can be used alone as a skin-softening mask for all skin types.

CONTRAINDICATIONS: Some people with extremely irritated, hypersensitive, sunburned, or windburned skin may experience discomfort and a stinging sensation from the lactic acid that naturally occurs in yogurt, but this is rare. Most of the time, yogurt counteracts the pain induced from environmental skin damage and helps speed healing of the condition.

THREE

Tools of the Trade for the Kitchen Cosmetologist

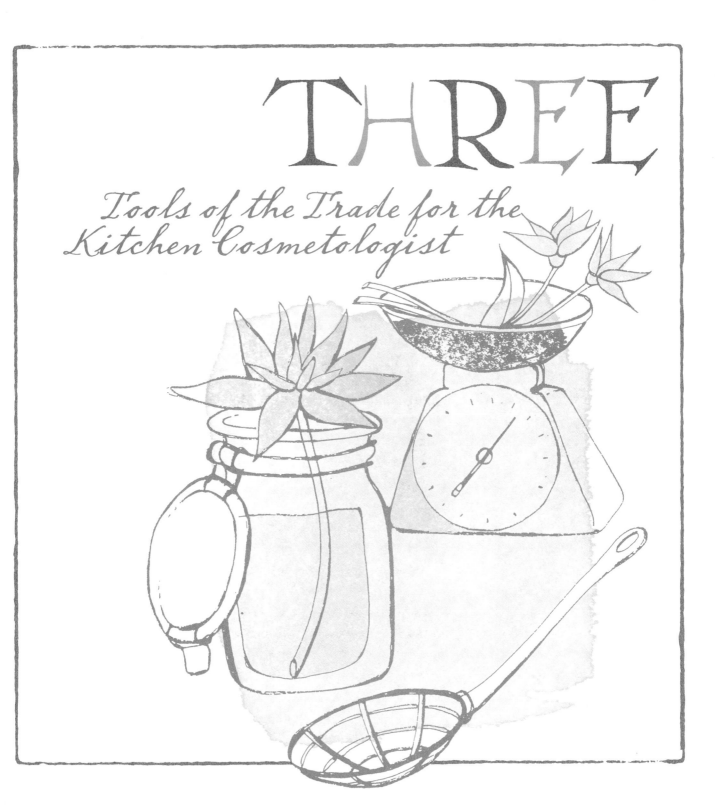

Making your own personal care products from natural ingredients is easy and soul-satisfying and can be a lot of fun. Only basic kitchen equipment and cooking skills are necessary for producing wonderfully fresh, body-nurturing creations. If you can boil water and make homemade salad dressing or mayonnaise, oatmeal, or pudding, then putting together these recipes will be as easy as pie.

"Cleanliness is next to Godliness," as the saying goes, and whether you're preparing dinner for 12 or making personal care products, the same stringent sanitary precautions apply. Ideally, all implements necessary for formulation — pots, pans, spatulas, spoons, whisks, blender, knives, cutting board, storage containers, and every other tool — should be boiled or sterilized, but that's not practical or always possible. The next best alternative is to run through the dishwasher everything you'll be using or to soak implements for 15 minutes in very, very hot soapy water to which you've added one teaspoon of bleach for each gallon of water. Give them a good scrub and then dry them thoroughly. The goal: to minimize the potential for harmful bacterial growth in your preservative-free products.

I cannot emphasize enough that your containers need to be as sterile as possible, dry, and dust-free prior to pouring into them your newly made recipes, and that your hands should be just-washed and dried as well. Introducing the tiniest bit of bacteria into your product will cause mold to take hold quickly, especially when you've made a product that combines water or a water-based ingredient such as an herbal hydrosol, herbal infusion or tea, or aloe vera juice with an oil or solid fat, as is called for in some cream and lotion recipes. Within two weeks or less after the introduction of bacteria, your lovely, aromatic, skin-pampering concoction will sport greenish-gray, fuzzy growth and you'll have to pitch it. What a waste! As with any worthwhile project you pursue in life, proper preparation is key!

Three lists are included in this chapter. The first includes equipment needed for preparing your personal care recipes; the second covers storage container options based on which work best with a particular product; and the third includes applicators and cleansing tools, identifying some common and not-so-common items that will ensure that you get the most from your creations.

Preparation Tools

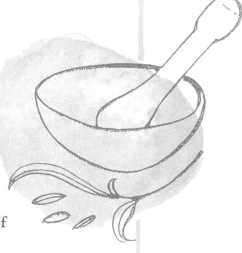

Common, easy-to-find kitchen tools are all you need to make the body care recipes in this book. Regarding quality, inexpensive tools will likely wear out quickly and have to be replaced. Generally, middle-of-the-road quality is fine (unless you want to indulge yourself and purchase a top-of-the-line blender or coffee grinder for your projects). Here's a list of what you'll need.

- **Blender.** This is great for whipping together creams and lotions in quantities of 2 cups or more. When mixing smaller quantities, I find it difficult to get all the cream or lotion out of the bottom of the blender. A blender can also be used to grind oatmeal, almonds, and sunflower seeds into meal, but a food processor or nut or seed grinder usually works much better.
- **Bowls.** You'll need a variety of sizes in glass, enamel, plastic, stainless steel, or ceramic. I use small bowls for mixing masks, single-serving facial scrubs, nail conditioners, and dentifrices, and larger bowls for mixing the ingredients for herbal facial steams and body powders or making anything in quantity for myself or gift giving. Occasionally I use plastic, lidded bowls for dry storage. Don't use them if you've previously used them to store tomato sauce or anything

strongly flavored; plastic tends to absorb odors and flavors and can leach these into your products.

- **Cheesecloth.** You'll use this for straining herbs from liquids and for making bath and wash bags. A nylon stocking or coarsely woven burlap make good substitutes, though coffee filters are my preferred choice for filtering watery liquids.

- **Coffee filters.** I like to use the small or medium filters as liners for my mesh strainers so that I can remove all particulate matter (when desired) from herbal infusions or teas and herbal infused oils. Simply insert a coffee filter into your strainer and pour your liquid. Perfectly clean herbal infusions will strain through.

- **Coffee grinder.** This kitchen gadget gets more use than any other piece of equipment I own aside from my blender. It's basically the same as a nut or seed grinder. I grind oatmeal, almonds, sunflower seeds, and dried flowers to the precise texture I want. Be sure to use separate grinders for your personal care products and your coffee! Coffee beans leave a lingering flavor and aroma in the grinder that will permeate your natural cosmetic ingredients, thereby tainting your creations.

- **Cutting board.** Made of either wood or plastic (choose your favorite material), this item is used for slicing and dicing miscellaneous items. Always keep a separate board for processing any dairy, meat, poultry, or fish products. Remember to keep your boards scrupulously clean at all times; they can harbor bacteria in grooved and sliced areas.

- **Double boiler.** This consists of one pan set inside another of the same size. Some manufacturers specifically make double boiler pans using this arrangement. To use the pan, fill the bottom pan with water that will come to a boil, thus heating the base of the top pan. I occasionally use a double boiler to melt hard or thick ingredients, such as wax, cocoa butter, shea butter, or coconut oil, and to warm liquid oils when making various creams, lotions, and lip balms. The advantage of this tool is that it produces a gentle, even, relatively low heat, making it impossible to scorch or boil your ingredients if you happen to get called away from the kitchen or get distracted. Usually, though, I simply choose a basic stainless steel pan (or pans), and use the low setting on my stove to melt and warm my ingredients, stirring occasionally.

Note: When making products that contain fatty ingredients such as oils, waxes, or butters, low heat is the key. If you simmer, overheat, boil, or scorch these ingredients, they'll be ruined. In this case, the saying "a watched pot never boils" is a good thing! In making body care products, always keep a watchful eye on what you're doing.

- **Eyedropper (glass).** Use this for measuring essential oils by the drop. Glass is preferable because unlike plastic, it doesn't retain scent or color from other essential oils you measure, and some essential oils, especially citrus oils, can actually degrade plastic and rubber. After each use, rinse the dropper with hot water, then pour isopropyl rubbing alcohol through it to sterilize it or boil it in distilled water. Allow the dropper to dry completely before using it again.

- **Food processor (full-sized or small model).** This can be used for mixing larger amounts (usually 4 cups or more) of creams and lotions, face and body scrubs, facial masks, and body powders, or for making finely ground oatmeal, almond meal, and sunflower seed meal.

- **Funnel (plastic or stainless steel).** This comes in handy when pouring liquid recipes into narrow-necked storage bottles. If you don't have this actual item, a funnel can be made from aluminum foil in a snap, and because herbal liquids pass through a funnel so quickly, there is no real risk of aluminum leaching into your product, as there is with using aluminum pots and pans.
- **Measuring cups and spoons.** Preparing creams and lotions frequently requires exact measurements, which is where these come in handy. Glass, plastic, or stainless steel is fine. If you like the convenience of a microwave, some herbalists I know use incrementally marked glass measuring cups (or bowls) in the microwave (versus pots on a stovetop) to warm and melt all their ingredients. Glass measuring cups or bowls of this kind are easy to hold (most have a handle), and because of the easy-to-read measurement markings, you can be sure you've measured ingredients accurately. Product perfection is virtually guaranteed — as long as you don't overheat the ingredients!
- **Mortar and pestle (large-sized, with a mortar approximately 6 inches in diameter).** I use this tool to crush fennel seeds; crush fresh herbs and flowers to extract their juices; and mash ripe papaya, banana, pineapple chunks, or ripe berries. A mortar and pestle is also handy for combining essential oils and unscented powder mixtures for herbal body powders.
- **Pans.** I use myriad sizes that vary from a tiny, ¾-quart pan to 1-, 2-, 3-, and 6-quart enamel, glass, or stainless steel pans. Please do not use aluminum or copper pans. These metals can react with the herbs, fruits, resins, and acid liquids in your recipes and leach the aluminum and copper

into the products you're making. Aluminum, in particular, is not good for your skin. It can also affect the beneficial qualities of the herbs and can discolor the end product.

- **Paring knives.** Always keep several very sharp blades at your disposal for cutting and peeling just about anything. I cut or shave beeswax with a paring knife instead of using a cheese grater. It's easier on my knuckles!

- **Scale (tabletop or diet model).** When I first began making personal care products, I used my scale constantly. Now, I can usually judge by sight the amount of an ingredient I'm measuring. A scale is not a necessity, but it's nice to have if you like to know how much your final product weighs. In this book, I don't use ounces as measurements in my recipes, so you can get away without purchasing one. It can be eye-opening, however, to see how much space 4 ounces of dried rose petals takes up compared to 4 ounces of dried comfrey root! A scale is a good learning tool for the beginner.

- **Spatulas (small and medium).** These are perfect for scooping out creams, lotions, balms, salves, and butters from any type of container. I find that long-handled, narrow spatulas come in handy when I need to occasionally free up the oil- and wax-clogged blender blades as I mix thick creams and lotions.

- **Spoons (wooden).** You really need only two: one small and one medium-sized. These should suffice for everything that needs stirring. If my whisk is dirty, I'll use a spoon to whip small quantities of creams and lotions. They're indispensable. *Note:* A stainless steel iced teaspoon works well for blending and whipping liquids in tiny pans if you don't have a wooden one handy.

- Strainer (bamboo, wire, or fabric mesh). Use this to strain herbs and flowers from liquids in various recipes. Cheesecloth, a nylon stocking, a coffee filter, or burlap can be used as substitutes.
- Whisks (small and large). I use the small one for whipping and blending creams, lotions, and lip and body balms. It works best for blending small amounts, while the blender or food processor work better for larger recipes. I use a large whisk for gently stirring body powder blends or larger quantities of body and facial scrubs.

2 Tablespoons = 1 Ounce
Math and Kitchen Cosmetology

Don't panic and bite your nails because the word *math* appears here! Whether you're a beginner or an experienced cosmetic cook, it's good to know a few simple measurement equivalents. Commit these to memory and they'll make preparation of your products a bit quicker, especially if you want to customize a recipe or make a larger or smaller batch than indicated in the recipe's yield.

BY THE TABLESPOON
⅓ tablespoon = 1 teaspoon
1 tablespoon = 3 teaspoons = ½ fluid ounce
2 tablespoons = 28 grams = 1 fluid ounce
4 tablespoons = ¼ cup = 2 fluid ounces
16 tablespoons = 1 cup = 8 ounces or ½ pint

BY THE OUNCE
1 ounce = 28 grams
8 ounces = 1 cup
16 ounces = 2 cups = 1 pint
32 ounces = 4 cups = 2 pints or 1 quart
1 gallon = 16 cups = 4 quarts

Storage Containers

The more attractive and user-friendly the containers for storing your hand-made personal care products, the better. Remember that many high-end cosmetics are packaged in containers that cost more than the ingredients they contain! Aesthetic appeal is important — especially if you intend to give your products as gifts. See Resources for mail-order companies that sell storage containers, or frequent antique shops and flea markets for unusual and one-of-a-kind ornamental bottles, jars, and tins. For these special products, a recycled mustard jar will not do! Here are some storage container ideas.

- **Bottles (½ ounce to 16 ounces).** I use dark glass and plastic. These are great for storing anything liquid, from astringents and toners to shampoos, bath and massage oils, and mouthwashes. If using glass, choose brown, green, or blue, especially if the product will be exposed to bright light for an extended period of time. Dark glass helps preserve the volatile natural properties of herbs, base oils, and essential oils. When traveling or if your home is full of small children and pets, plastic bottles might be preferable. Just be sure to store them away from light once filled.
- **Canning jars (½ pint to 1 gallon).** These are suitable for storing dried herbs away from light and for making solar-infused oils. The half-pint size is perfect for packaging scrubs, masks, and dry herbal cleansers to give to friends. Slap on your custom label and voilà! you've got a beautiful present!

- Cream jars (¼ ounce to 8 ounces). These are perfect for creams, lip and body balms, healing salves, bath salts, and face and body scrubs. These jars are available in glass or plastic.
- Muslin bags. These are available in a variety of sizes, or you can sew your own custom size. They're useful for making bath bags, herbal sleep pillows, or large quantities of herbal "bath tea."
- Plastic tubs. Plastic food storage containers with airtight lids are available in grocery stores or through home product demonstrations. I use all sizes to store dried herbs, dry face and body cleansers and scrubs, masks, bath salts, and body powder blends.
- Shaker jars (glass or plastic). Use these types of jars for herbal body powders. The grocery store I frequent sells generic spices in 2½-inch diameter, 2¼-ounce plastic shaker containers. After using the spice, I wash these thoroughly and save them for my powders. I sometimes store dry face and body scrub mixtures in them as well.
- Spritzer bottles (glass or plastic). These are good for packaging astringents, toners, and insect repellents — or any recipe that requires a spray application.
- Squeeze bottles. These plastic bottles are great storage containers for shampoos, conditioners, bath oils and massage oils, astringents, and toners.
- Tins (¼ ounce to 8 ounce or larger). Tins have a lovely, old-fashioned appeal and look very attractive when decorated with a custom-made label, making them great gift-giving containers. I like to use these to store dried herbs, body powders with a fancy puff, dry cleansers, and dry face and body scrubs. They also make perfect travel containers

for small portions of sleep and headache-relieving balms. They're relatively airtight and keep out both bugs and light.

- Woozys. Beautiful, decorative glass bottles designed mainly for culinary use as wine and vinegar containers, these narrow-necked, tall bottles are super for storing face and body splashes, floral waters, and bath and massage oils. They're also perfect for gift giving.

- Zip-seal freezer bags. These make terrific storage containers for dry scrubs or cleansers, bath salts, dry body scrub bases, or excess body powder if you've made a large quantity. You can also store dried herbs for months in these bags if you keep them in a dry, cool, dark place.

RECYCLING STORAGE CONTAINERS

If you plan to recycle previously used glass, plastic, or ceramic containers for storage purposes, please be sure to wash them thoroughly first. You can either run them through the dishwasher or allow them to soak for 15 minutes in very hot, soapy water with a splash of added bleach. After they've soaked, scrub thoroughly, rinse, and allow them to dry completely. Do not store your cosmetics in containers that have previously held medicine, poisons, household cleansers (other than dishwashing liquid), spoiled foods, or fertilizers. Use your own good judgment about what containers *are* and *are not* safe to use.

Application and Cleansing Tools

The following is a list of handy-to-have items that make application and removal of many personal care products more effective and enjoyable. These items are not required, but all are useful.

- **Complexion brush.** These brushes are usually about the size of your palm or may have a short handle with the bristles forming a 1- to 1½-inch diameter circular pattern at the end. The bristles should be very, very soft, akin to an infant's hairbrush, and can be either synthetic or natural. Use a complexion brush much as you would a washcloth, but steer clear of the eye area. Store your brush in such a way that it will dry thoroughly between uses. A consistently damp brush will encourage mold growth and will destroy the area where the bristles attach to the base. Be sure to give the brush a thorough washing with soap and water at least once per week.

- **Cosmetic fan brush.** This is a slender-handled cosmetic brush approximately 6 inches to 8 inches long, with fan-shaped natural or synthetic bristles. Estheticians frequently use these brushes to "paint" masks onto the face for even distribution or to apply thinned yogurt or fruit pulp. They are available from better drug and beauty supply stores.

- **Cotton balls or cotton squares.** There are so many uses for these I can't mention them all here. I like to soak them in cold milk or herb tea and apply them as soothing eye pads or soak them with oil to remove stubborn eye makeup. Many people use them to apply astringent or toner or moisten them with cleanser to gently cleanse the face and neck. I prefer to buy 100 percent cotton balls or squares or cut my own from rolled cotton sometimes called "beautician's cotton." Rolled cotton can be purchased from your local beauty supply store.

- **Facial shammy cloth.** This is a synthetic version of a washcloth — about the same size, rather thin, slightly rubbery, and very soft. I highly recommend it for cleansing ultrasensitive, acneic, or environmentally damaged skin. It makes a perfect cloth for the delicate skin of an infant or very thin, papery, elderly skin.

- **Loofah sponge.** A loofah is actually the dried skeleton of a gourd. Available at most health food and drug stores, it's excellent for daily exfoliation of dry skin buildup on the body but is too rough for use on the face. Like a sponge, a loofah is wonderful to use with foaming body cleansers. Loofahs tend to retain moisture and can mold easily, so after use, be sure to place your damp sponge in an upright position where it can dry and receive plenty of air circulation.

- **Sea sponge (tiny, medium, or large).** Many women like to use small sea sponges for face cleansing and the larger ones in the bath or shower when applying foaming cleansers. *Remember:* A little foaming cleanser goes a long way when applied with a sponge versus a washcloth. Like loofah sponges, these can mold easily. Please find a storage place where they can dry between uses.

- Tissues. Men often wonder why women go through so many tissues. Well, some of us use them for everything under the sun, including to blot excess perspiration and oil from the face, to blot or remove lipstick, and to remove cleansing creams and lotions and eye makeup when a washcloth is unavailable. If you're in need of either invigoration or relaxation, place a few drops of the appropriate essential oil onto a tissue and inhale as needed or tuck it into your blouse or under your pillow at night. Use only unscented, white tissues — dyes and deodorants may irritate delicate skin. For cosmetic purposes, avoid ultrasoft, puffy, lotion-impregnated tissues, which can be very fibrous and can leave tiny bits of annoying fuzz on your face and lips.
- Washing puff or cleansing pad. This soft, often white pad is usually a circular piece of 3- or 5-inch foam covered with fine-textured terry cloth. It works just like a washcloth, but tends to be less fibrous and is thus gentler on the skin.

FOUR

All-Natural Face and Body Care Recipes

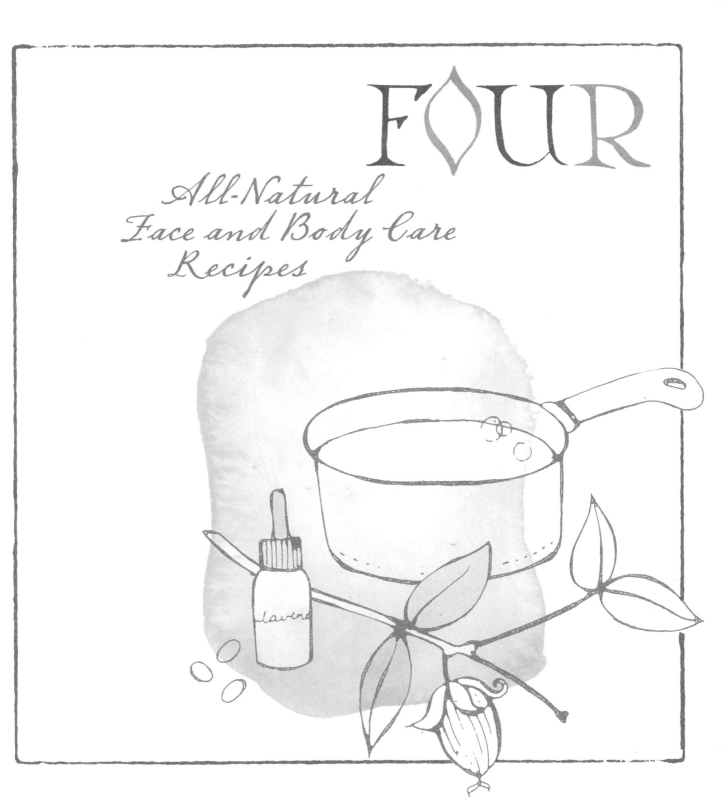

In a culinary cookbook, we primarily use a recipe as a road map, which, if we follow it correctly, will lead us to a delicious destination. But a food recipe can be so much more than this. It can sometimes offer us a glimpse of history or a view into current cultural trends, or it can share tidbits of interesting nutritional knowledge. The ingredients in a recipe often let us see into the soul of the individual cook.

Personal care recipes are somewhat similar. If you've ever delved into the history of fashion, hygiene, and health from, say, the 1600s to the early 1900s, you've doubtless come across books that describe the particular natural ingredients people used to heal cuts and bruises; cure the common cold; cleanse, deodorize, and perfume their bodies and homes; and beautify their face and hair. Such books open a window into the world of natural personal care before the chemical age of synthetics.

In this chapter, you'll find my favorite tried-and-true formulas for making natural personal care products for the face, body, eyes, lips, hands, feet, and mouth. Unlike formulas of the past, these recipes incorporate the use of new blending equipment, ingredient extraction technologies, preservation methods, and a wider array of ingredients available today — all of which allow homemade formulas to rival many commercially available products, sans synthetics.

Before we begin, it's important to note a few points about the recipes themselves:

- All herbs called for are in *dried* form unless otherwise specified.
- Each ingredient is included in a recipe for a specific reason — it contributes to the integrity of the final product.
- As your knowledge of personal care products grows and you gain valuable blending experience, I encourage you to use the recipes here more as guidelines so that you can customize some to suit your personal specifications. As your skills develop, experiment and add your own special touch to each.

Be creative and enjoy the process!

Face Care

There are several steps to take and products from which to choose in order to properly care for and pamper the face and its often neglected associated areas, the neck and décolleté (upper chest). The following formulas includes recipes for many types of cleansers, refreshing agents, masks, herbal steams, exfoliants, traditional moisturizers and new emollient elixirs, eye treatments, lip balms, and oral hygiene. Simply choose the ones that suit your current skin type and particular needs, keeping in mind your environment and lifestyle habits.

Face Cleansers

Regardless of the type, cleansers are designed to remove everyday dirt and grime that collects in your facial pores. Creamy and oil-based cleansers, however, do a better job of removing makeup than foaming, powdered, or clay-based products and are frequently used as an initial makeup cleanser, followed by a second cleansing with the same product or with a foaming liquid, solid mild soap, clay-based cleanser, or powdered soap-free cleanser. All of these recipes are very gentle, nourishing, and do a thorough job of cleansing.

"COOKING" TIPS: Several of the following recipes require the heating and melting of various oils, waxes, butters, and water-based ingredients for blending. When "cooking" your cleansing creams, please use the *low* setting on your stove to warm or melt the ingredients in a saucepan or use a double boiler or the microwave. (If you choose to use the microwave, warm ingredients for only 10 to 15 seconds at a time to avoid overheating.) Whatever "cooking" method you choose, *never allow the herbal liquid or wax/oil/butter mixture to get too hot or bubble or simmer.* Gently warm them enough just for the solids to melt and the borax (when called for) to dissolve in the herbal liquid. To blend properly, the wax/oil/butter should be the same temperature as the herbal liquid/borax mixture, about body temperature or slightly cooler. Remember that blending takes a bit of practice. You're attempting to combine oil with water — which naturally repel each other — and get them to stabilize chemically and form an emulsion. Just as occurs with homemade mayonnaise or buttercream frosting, though, when water and oil are blended properly and at the right temperatures, magic happens! A fabulous cream appears right before your eyes.

CONSISTENCY TIPS: To make a cream thicker or firmer, add a tad more beeswax, cocoa butter, or shea butter. Experiment and see which one produces the consistency and texture you like best. Shea butter will always remain softer than beeswax or cocoa butter.

STORAGE TIPS: The cleansing creams here contain no preservatives and thus have a short shelf life. They generally require no refrigeration if used completely within thirty days unless the weather is very hot. If cleansing cream is stored unopened in the refrigerator and the product is untouched, it may last up to six months. Please note that though refrigeration may change the product's texture, it will not affect its potency. Foaming, oil-based, and powdered cleansers need no refrigeration and generally have a much longer shelf life than cleansing creams and lotions. Specific refrigeration and storage requirements are included with each recipe.

SAFETY CONSIDERATIONS

Many of the recipes here will look and smell edible because the majority of ingredients used will be edible, but this does not mean that any particular product here is safe to consume. *Unless the recipe specifically states that it's edible (and a handful of flavored body balms are), do not eat the result!* Please, for safety's sake, clearly label all your personal care products and keep them out of the reach of children and pets.

If you are allergy-prone, it's best to test yourself for adverse reactions to the herbs called for in any recipe you're planning to use. To do this, use *a patch test:* Prepare a paste with ½ teaspoon of the herb in question and a small amount of boiling water, and then apply the paste to *cleansed* skin on the inside of your elbow. Cover with an adhesive bandage and leave on for 12 to 24 hours.

If you're concerned about a potential allergic reaction to an essential oil, dilute 1 or 2 drops with 1 teaspoon of bland vegetable oil such as soybean or olive oil, saturate a cotton ball with the mixture, and apply in the same way and in the same place as the paste.

To test any other ingredient, simply apply a small amount to the same spot on your arm and cover with a bandage for the same amount of time. If a rash or redness appears, *do not* use this ingredient. Substitute another that causes no reaction. (See the Ingredient Dictionary in chapter 2 for possible substitutes.)

While making your personal care products, if any of the solutions or mixtures enter your eye or eyes, promptly flood them with an unscented, bland fatty oil such as almond, olive, corn, soybean, peanut, or generic vegetable oil (in the case of essential oil accidents), water, or cold milk repeatedly. If any irritation continues, see your health care provider as soon as possible.

ALOE AND CALENDULA CLEANSING CREAM

*T*his cleansing cream removes makeup, dirt, and grime, and has powerful moisturizing, hydrating, and anti-inflammatory properties. It's soothing to damaged
skin and doubles as a fabulous face and body cream and after-sun treatment. If you're
using it as a face moisturizer, you'll need only a pea-sized dollop of product. Use it as
needed for the body.

¼ cup almond, sunflower,
    or soybean base oil
2   tablespoons coconut base oil
    (extra-virgin, unrefined)
2   tablespoons beeswax
1   teaspoon anhydrous lanolin
¼   cup pure aloe vera juice
3   tablespoons strong calendula
    blossom or chamomile flower
    tea (you can substitute distilled
    water or your favorite hydrosol)
1   tablespoon vegetable glycerin
¼   teaspoon borax
1   large or 2 small vitamin E
    oil capsules
15 drops lavender essential oil
15 drops rosemary
    (chemotype *verbenon*) or
    geranium essential oil
8   drops calendula essential oil
    (CO2 extract), (optional)

RECOMMENDED FOR: *normal, dry,
mature, sensitive, or environmentally
damaged skin*
USE: *daily*
FOLLOW WITH: *astringent or toner*
PREP TIME: *approximately 20 to 30
minutes, plus 30 minutes to cool and
set up*
BLENDING TOOLS: *blender, spoon*
STORE IN: *glass or plastic jars*
YIELD: *approximately 1 cup*

HEAT: In a small saucepan over low heat or in a double boiler,
warm the base oils, beeswax, and lanolin until the wax is just melted.
In another pan, lightly warm the aloe vera juice, tea, and vegetable
glycerin, and stir in the borax until it dissolves in the liquid.

COOL: Remove both pans from heat and pour the oils/wax/lanolin mixture into the blender and allow it to cool until it just begins to thicken and becomes slightly opaque. It will be like a soft, loose salve. This will take approximately 5 to 10 minutes, depending on the temperature of your kitchen. As it thickens, give the mixture a few stirs to remove any lumps and incorporate any of the mixture that sticks to the sides of the blender. Do not allow this mixture to get too thick or you may have a difficult time getting it out of your blender.

BLEND: Place the lid on the blender and remove the lid's plastic piece. Turn the blender on high and slowly drizzle the watery juice/tea/glycerin/borax mixture through the center of the lid into the vortex of swirling fats below. Closely watch what happens: Almost immediately the cream will turn pale yellow and will begin to thicken. Blend for about 10 to 15 seconds until all the watery mixture has been added, then check the consistency of the cream. It should have a smooth texture. If the water mixture is not properly combining with the oils/wax/lanolin mixture, turn off the blender and give the cream a few manual stirs with a spatula to free up the blender blades. Then, replace the lid and blend on medium for another 5 to 10 seconds. Repeat this process until cream is smooth.

Pierce the vitamin E capsule(s) and squeeze the contents into the cream, add the essential oils, then blend completely another 5 seconds until the cream is smooth and thick.

Note: If the temperature of your kitchen is above 76°F, the cream will maintain a softer consistency. (Coconut oil turns from solid to liquid at 76°F). If your kitchen is below 76°F, the cream will be firmer.

PACKAGE AND COOL: Pour the finished cream into storage container(s). Lightly cover each container with a paper towel and allow the cream to cool for about 30 minutes before capping. If, after a few hours or days, water begins to separate from your cream, don't worry. You can pour off the watery liquid and use the resulting product as a foot, elbow, or knee balm. The mixture can separate if the fat temperature and water temperature are not relatively equal and cool enough when the two portions are blended.

No refrigeration is required if used within 30 days. If your storage area is very warm, please use within 3 weeks for maximum potency and freshness.

APPLICATION TIPS: Using a soft cloth, cleansing pad, or your fingers, apply approximately ½ to 1 teaspoon to cover entire face, throat, and décolleté.

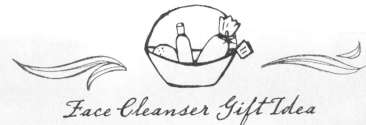

Face Cleanser Gift Idea

Freshly made face cleansers, along with an appropriate toner or astringent and moisturizer, make a complete skin care gift for a dear friend.

- Package cosmetics in glass containers such as French jelly jars or small cobalt blue jars or bottles.
- Label each product with a decorative sticker or personalized computer label.
- Line a small basket with a brightly colored face cloth, sprinkle a few tablespoons of lavender buds or rose petals in the bottom, and place your cosmetics.
- Tie a ribbon around the basket.
- Print complete instructions for each cosmetic on fine stationary or parchment paper and include it in an envelope or roll it as a scroll and tie it with a ribbon or raffia.

See Astringents and Toners: Refreshing Agents on page 127 for suggestions on how to bottle herbal tonics.

BASIC COLD CREAM AND MAKEUP REMOVER

I use this primarily as a makeup remover for heavy stage makeup, but it doubles as a terrific ultra-thick moisturizing foot and "flaky shin" cream.

1 tablespoon jojoba base oil

7 tablespoons pure vegetable shortening (No lard, please!)

10 drops lavender or Roman chamomile essential oil

RECOMMENDED FOR: *normal, dry, sensitive, mature, or environmentally damaged skin*
USE: *daily*
FOLLOW WITH: *astringent or toner*
PREP TIME: *approximately 20 to 30 minutes, plus 1 to 2 hours to set up*
BLENDING TOOLS: *small spoon or whisk*
STORE IN: *plastic or glass jar*
YIELD: *½ cup*

In a small saucepan over low heat or in a double boiler, warm the oil and shortening until the two have completely melted. Remove from heat and allow to cool for 5 to 10 minutes. Add the essential oil, then begin stirring slowly with a small spoon or whisk until the mixture begins to thicken and become opaque. Pour into storage jars and cap.

Depending on the temperature of your working space, the product may take a couple of hours to completely set up and attain its thick, creamy consistency. If you wish to hasten this, you can place container(s) in the refrigerator for 30 minutes. No refrigeration of the finished product is required, but for maximum freshness and potency, please use within 6 to 12 months.

APPLICATION TIPS: Using a soft cloth, cleansing pad, or your fingers, apply approximately ½ to 1 teaspoon to cover entire face, throat, and décolleté.

Herbal Soapy Skin Wash

This product doubles as an especially invigorating body wash for oily and normal skin and also makes an effective antibacterial hand soap. It's excellent for use on back acne and as a shampoo for oily hair (if diluted 50 percent with distilled or purified water).

1   16-ounce bottle unscented liquid castile soap

5   drops **each** of the following essential oils: tea tree; peppermint; green myrtle; German chamomile

1   teaspoon hazelnut or jojoba base oil

RECOMMENDED FOR: *oily, acneic, combination, or normal skin*
USE: *daily*
FOLLOW WITH: *astringent or toner*
PREP TIME: *approximately 10 minutes*
BLENDING TOOLS: *shake before each use*
STORE IN: *castile soap bottle*
YIELD: *approximately 2 cups*

Add the essential oils and teaspoon of base oil to the bottle of castile soap. Shake vigorously. Store the finished product right in the castile soap bottle.

No refrigeration is required, but for maximum freshness and potency, please use within 1 year.

APPLICATION TIPS: Shake the mixture well and using a soft cloth, cleansing pad, or your fingers, apply approximately ½ to 1 teaspoon to cover entire face, throat, and décolleté. *Remember:* Castile soap is highly concentrated, so a little goes a long way. Rinse.

EVER-SO-GENTLE SOAP LOVER'S FLORAL FACE AND BODY WASH

This recipe dilutes the castile soap by 50 percent with skin-pampering hydrosols, thus creating a very gentle liquid soap product for virtually all skin types. It's perfect for those who insist on using soap and makes an effective, floral-scented, calming cleanser for the entire body. I like to use this formula when my normal-to-dry skin becomes seasonally oily in the summer.

1   8-ounce bottle unscented liquid castile soap
½   cup neroli hydrosol
½   cup rose geranium hydrosol
1   teaspoon jojoba oil
10   drops geranium essential oil
10   drops neroli essential oil (optional)

RECOMMENDED FOR: *all skin types except very dry, dehydrated, or environmentally damaged skin*
USE: *daily*
FOLLOW WITH: *astringent or toner*
PREP TIME: *approximately 10 minutes*
BLENDING TOOLS: *shake well before each use*
STORE IN: *plastic squeeze bottle or glass bottle*
YIELD: *approximately 2 cups*

Add all ingredients to a 2-cup or larger plastic container. Shake or stir well to blend.

Pour into storage container(s), preferably plastic squeeze bottles.

No refrigeration is required, but for maximum freshness and potency, please use within 1 year.

APPLICATION TIPS: Using a soft cloth, cleansing pad, or your fingers, apply approximately 1 teaspoon to cover entire face, throat, and décolleté (or more as necessary for use on the body). Shake well before each use.

Minty Soap Lover's Face and Body Wash

This recipe dilutes the castile soap by 50 percent with distilled water and wonderfully fragrant, highly anti-inflammatory lemon balm hydrosol, thus creating a very gentle liquid soap product for virtually all skin types. It's perfect for mint lovers and for those who insist on using soap and makes an effective, invigorating, aromatic, pick-me-up cleanser for the entire body.

1   8-ounce bottle unscented liquid castile soap
½   cup lemon balm hydrosol
½   cup distilled water
1   teaspoon jojoba oil
10   drops spearmint essential oil
10   drops peppermint essential oil

RECOMMENDED FOR: *all skin types except very dry, dehydrated, or environmentally damaged skin*
USE: *daily*
FOLLOW WITH: *astringent or toner*
PREP TIME: *approximately 10 minutes*
BLENDING TOOLS: *shake before each use*
STORE IN: *plastic squeeze bottle or glass bottle*
YIELD: *approximately 2 cups*

Add all ingredients to a 2-cup or larger plastic container. Shake or stir well to blend.

Pour into storage container(s), preferably plastic squeeze bottles.

No refrigeration is required, but for maximum freshness and potency, please use within 1 year.

APPLICATION TIPS: Using a soft cloth, cleansing pad, or your fingers, apply approximately 1 teaspoon to cover entire face, throat, and décolleté (or more as necessary for use on the body). Shake well before each use.

LAVENDER AND ROSES GENTLE CLEANSER

*T*his is a delicately fragranced cleanser for those who don't wear much facial makeup. It will not spoil as long as you don't let moisture enter the container and it makes a good multiuse product. It can double as a face mask and gentle exfoliant; spread it on cleansed skin and let it dry for 20 minutes.

½ cup white clay, finely ground

⅓ cup ground oatmeal or oat flour

1 tablespoon powdered lavender buds

1 tablespoon powdered rose petals

5 drops lavender essential oil

2 drops rose otto or geranium essential oil

RECOMMENDED FOR: *all skin types*
USE: *daily*
FOLLOW WITH: *astringent or toner*
PREP TIME: *10 to 15 minutes*
BLENDING TOOLS: *plastic bag*
STORE IN: *plastic or glass jar, tin, or plastic bag*
YIELD: *approximately 1 cup*

Place all ingredients except the essential oils into a plastic bag. Secure bag opening with a twist tie or zip-seal the top to close. Shake well to blend, then add the essential oils by the drop, close the bag, and shake again.

Pour the product into a storage container or leave it in the plastic bag.

No refrigeration is required, but for maximum freshness and potency, please store in a cool, dry place and use within 6 months.

TO MIX THE CLEANSER FOR USE: Place 2 teaspoons of powdered cleanser into a small bowl (or the palm of your hand) and add 2 teaspoons of water, milk, or cream. Stir to blend until a spreadable paste forms, and allow this paste to thicken 1 minute.

APPLICATION TIPS: Using a soft cloth, cleansing pad, or your fingers, apply entire mixture to cover face, throat, and décolleté (avoiding the eye area) and massage in circular motions for 1 minute. Rinse.

CLEANSING AND REJUVENATING OIL

This product is an excellent makeup remover, but follow with a second cleansing using this oil or another cleanser of your choice to ensure that skin is deep-down clean. This unique oil blend nourishes dry, parched skin and maintains the glow of normal, healthy skin. Oily skin can benefit from the vitamin- and mineral-rich oils, too, but make sure to apply the appropriate astringent following cleansing to remove any oil residue. This blend can also be used as a face and body massage oil, bath oil, or as "skin food" for normal and dry skin (applied before bedtime and left on overnight in lieu of regular moisturizer).

2 tablespoons each almond, apricot kernel, avocado or sunflower seed, and extra-virgin olive base oil

1 large or 2 small vitamin E oil capsules

20 drops sweet orange, lavender, or neroli essential oil

RECOMMENDED FOR: *all skin types*
USE: *daily*
FOLLOW WITH: *astringent or toner*
PREP TIME: *approximately 10 to 15 minutes*
BLENDING TOOLS: *shake well before each use*
STORE IN: *plastic squirt bottle or glass bottle*
YIELD: *approximately ½ cup*

Combine the base oils in a storage container. Shake well to blend. Pierce the vitamin E capsule(s) and add to the mix. Add the essential oils, and shake again.

No refrigeration is required, but for maximum freshness and potency, please use within 6 months.

APPLICATION TIPS: Shake well before each use. Using a soft cloth, cleansing pad, or your fingers, apply approximately ½ to 1 teaspoon to cover entire face, throat, and décolleté (or more as necessary for use on the body).

Classic Rosewater and Glycerin Anytime Freshening Cleanser

This product does not remove makeup; with its old-fashioned, classic floral scent, it's best to use as a light, freshening cleanser on your makeup-free days or after playing sports. It doubles as a moisturizing toner for parched skin — it's very gentle and soothing and leaves skin feeling soft and smelling fragrant.

¾ cup rose hydrosol
¼ cup vegetable glycerin

RECOMMENDED FOR: *normal, dry, mature, sensitive, dehydrated, environmentally damaged, sunburned, or windburned skin*
USE: *daily*
FOLLOW WITH: *moisturizer if desired*
PREP TIME: *approximately 10 minutes*
BLENDING TOOLS: *shake well before each use*
STORE IN: *plastic or glass bottle or spritzer*
YIELD: *1 cup*

Combine ingredients in a storage container. Shake vigorously for about 30 seconds to blend.

No refrigeration is required, but for maximum freshness and potency, please use within 6 to 12 months.

APPLICATION TIPS: Use 1 teaspoon per application and apply this liquid cleanser with a washcloth or cleansing pad anytime your skin needs freshening.

LEMONY WHIP CLEANSING CREAM

Yes, you can use an oil-based, cleansing cream to cleanse oily and combination skin. Remember: Like removes like! The oils in the cream will actually dissolve and breakdown the dirty oils and makeup on your skin. If you feel that your skin needs additional cleansing, follow with a second cleansing using this same product or a dry, powdered, or liquid soapy cleanser.

¼ cup plus 3 tablespoons hazelnut or apricot kernel base oil

1 tablespoon coconut base oil (extra-virgin, unrefined)

1 tablespoon beeswax

1 teaspoon anhydrous lanolin

½ cup distilled water or lemon balm hydrosol

¼ teaspoon borax

1 large or 2 small vitamin E oil capsules

20 drops lemon essential oil

10 drops sweet orange essential oil

RECOMMENDED FOR: *oily, combination, or normal skin*
USE: *daily*
FOLLOW WITH: *astringent or toner*
PREP TIME: *approximately 20 to 30 minutes, plus 30 minutes to cool and set up*
BLENDING TOOLS: *blender*
STORE IN: *plastic or glass jars*
YIELDS: *approximately 1 cup*

HEAT: In a small saucepan over low heat or in a double boiler, warm the base oils, beeswax, and lanolin until the wax is just melted. In another pan, slightly warm the water or hydrosol and stir in the borax until it dissolves.

COOL: Remove both pans from heat and pour the oils/wax/lanolin mixture into the blender to cool until it just begins to thicken and becomes opaque, about 5 to 10 minutes. It will be a soft, loose salve. Give the mixture a few stirs to remove any lumps and incorporate any of the mixture that sticks to the sides of the blender.

BLEND: Place the lid on the blender and remove the lid's plastic piece. Turn the blender on high and slowly drizzle the water or hydrosol through the center of the lid into the vortex of swirling fats below. Closely watch what happens: Almost immediately the cream will turn pale yellow-gold and begin to thicken. Blend for about 10 to 15 seconds, adding all of the water or hydrosol, then check the consistency of the cream. It should have a smooth texture. If the water mixture is not properly combining with the oils/wax/lanolin mixture, turn off the blender and give the cream a few manual stirs with a spatula to free up the blades. Then replace the lid and blend on medium for 5 to 10 seconds. Repeat this process until the cream is smooth.

Pierce the vitamin E capsule(s) and squeeze the contents into the cream, add the essential oils, then blend completely another 5 seconds until the cream is smooth and thick.

Note: If the temperature of your kitchen is above 76°F, the cream will maintain a softer consistency. If your kitchen is below 76°F, the cream will be firmer.

PACKAGE AND COOL: Pour the finished cream into storage container(s). Lightly cover each container with a paper towel and allow the cream to cool for about 30 minutes before capping.

No refrigeration is required if used within 30 days. If your storage area is very warm, for maximum freshness and potency, please use within 3 weeks.

APPLICATION TIPS: Using a soft cloth, cleansing pad, or your fingers, apply approximately ½ to 1 teaspoon to cover entire face, throat, and décolleté. Rinse.

STRAWBERRY CLEANSER

S trawberry juice has gentle astringent and bleaching properties and is best used as a light cleanser for those who do not wear makeup. It can also serve as a tooth cleanser and whitener — it's very refreshing and helps eliminate onion and garlic breath.

4   very ripe, medium-sized strawberries, sliced and green stems removed
1   drop peppermint or lavender essential oil (optional)

RECOMMENDED FOR: *oily, combination, acneic, or normal skin*
USE: *daily when fresh strawberries are in season*
FOLLOW WITH: *astringent or toner*
PREP TIME: *5 to 10 minutes*
BLENDING TOOLS: *mortar and pestle or small bowl and fork*
STORE IN: *do not store; mix as needed*
YIELD: *1 application*

In a small bowl, thoroughly mash the strawberries with a fork (or use a mortar and pestle). Press the resulting pulp through a mesh strainer or squeeze through cheesecloth or nylon stocking and catch the juice in a small condiment bowl. Add the essential oil (if desired) and stir to blend.

APPLICATION TIPS: Apply juice to face, neck, and décolleté with a saturated cotton square (avoiding eye area), and massage with fingertips for about 1 minute. Rinse with cool water.

Astringents and Toners: Refreshing Agents

Astringents and toners are water-based agents used to remove cleanser residue, balance pH level, and hydrate the skin and are also effective at removing excess perspiration and oil.

Astringents tend to be stronger than toners and are usually used on oily, combination, and normal skin types. Many commercial astringents contain isopropyl alcohol and/or acetone (a strong, synthetic solvent found in nail polish removers), which are very drying and damaging to the skin. Herbal astringents, however, are gentle.

Toners, sometimes referred to as skin fresheners, perform the same function as an astringent but are designed for normal, dry, sensitive, dehydrated, mature, and environmentally damaged skin.

Remember that an aromatic hydrosol (see page 73) can always be used as a toner or gentle astringent. A bonus: Hydrosols do not require refrigeration.

STORAGE TIPS: Unless otherwise indicated, all of the following astringent and toner recipes should be stored in the refrigerator and used within 1 week to preserve freshness. Chemical preservatives are not used in these recipes to extend the shelf life of the product. Please store your products in tightly sealed and labeled bottles or spritzers.

APPLICATION TIPS: Always apply astringents and toners to the face and neck with a 100 percent cotton or silk-blend ball or pad using upward and outward strokes. Always follow the use of these products with an appropriate moisturizer for your skin type.

LEMON REFRESHER

The tart, lemony aroma of this astringent is very refreshing and stimulating to use chilled on a hot, summer day. Avoid use on sensitive, dehydrated, environmentally damaged, sunburned, windburned, or irritated skin.

Juice of half a medium-
    sized lemon,
    strained
½ cup witch hazel

RECOMMENDED FOR: *oily, combination, normal, or oily mature skin*
USE: *daily*
FOLLOW WITH: *moisturizer*
PREP TIME: *approximately 5 to 10 minutes*
BLENDING TOOLS: *shake before each use*
STORE IN: *plastic or glass bottle or spritzer*
YIELD: *approximately ½ cup*

Combine ingredients in a storage container and shake well to blend.

No refrigeration is required, but please use within 1 to 2 weeks, then discard.

APPLICATION TIPS: Using a cotton cleansing pad, apply approximately 1 teaspoon to the face or more to the shoulders or back as needed throughout the day. Avoid eye area.

Astringent and Toner Gift Idea

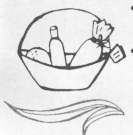

- Package one of your freshly made herbal astringents or toners in a colored glass or decorative woozy bottle.
- To make it even more enticing, add to the bottle a fresh sprig or peel of the herb called for in the recipe. Top it off with a decorative label stating the expiration date and a note on how to store and apply the product.

Parsley and Peppermint Astringent

This strong, green herbal infusion makes a gentle, yet powerful astringent to use on those days when your skin feels particularly hot and greasy, and is wonderful for use during hot flashes. It effectively removes excess oil without causing dryness.

2	cups distilled water
¼	cup fresh, chopped parsley
¼	cup fresh, chopped peppermint leaves
5	drops peppermint essential oil (optional)

RECOMMENDED FOR: *oily, acneic, combination, or normal skin*
USE: *daily*
FOLLOW WITH: *moisturizer*
PREP TIME: *approximately 35 minutes*
BLENDING TOOLS: *shake before each use*
STORE IN: *plastic or glass bottle or spritzer*
YIELD: *approximately 2 cups*

In a small saucepan, bring the water to boil and remove from heat. Add the herbs, cover, and allow to steep for 30 minutes. Add the essential oil (if desired), and stir to blend. Strain into storage container(s). Shake well.

Refrigerate for up to 1 week, then discard.

APPLICATION TIPS: Using a cotton cleansing pad, apply approximately 1 teaspoon to the face or more as necessary to the shoulders or back. Avoid eye area.

Astringent pH Restorer

The vinegar in this astringent will help combat the alkaline residue that soap or other cleansers can leave behind. When your skin maintains the correct pH balance, encouraged by this product, it has a much better chance of fighting off dryness and infections. This solution has a softening effect on the skin and doubles as a hair product: It effectively removes styling product buildup and enhances shine. Simply pour the entire recipe over hair after rinsing out conditioner. You can use this product weekly if desired.

2   cups distilled water
¼   cup raw apple cider vinegar
10   drops favorite essential oil (try lavender, lemon, or geranium)

RECOMMENDED FOR: *all skin types except sensitive, sunburned, windburned, irritated, or acneic (weeping) skin*
USE: *daily*
FOLLOW WITH: *moisturizer*
PREP TIME: *approximately 5 to 10 minutes*
BLENDING TOOLS: *shake before each use*
STORE IN: *plastic or glass bottle or spritzer*
YIELD: *approximately 2¼ cups*

Combine ingredients in a 3-cup or larger plastic container. Shake well to blend.

Pour into storage container(s).

No refrigeration is required, but for maximum freshness and potency, please use within 1 year.

APPLICATION TIPS: Using a cotton cleansing pad, apply approximately 1 teaspoon to the face or more as necessary if using as a body splash.

ACNE ASTRINGENT

This astringent is healing and soothing for weeping acne. It doubles as an effective healing wash for minor cuts and abrasions and also works well as a hair rinse if your scalp is oily.

2 cups distilled water

1 tablespoon yarrow

1 tablespoon calendula or chamomile flowers

6 drops juniper, rosemary (chemotype *verbenon*), or peppermint essential oil

RECOMMENDED FOR: *oily, combination, acneic, or normal skin*
USE: *daily*
FOLLOW WITH: *moisturizer*
PREP TIME: *approximately 35 minutes*
BLENDING TOOLS: *shake well before use*
STORE IN: *plastic or glass bottle or spritzer*
YIELD: *approximately 2 cups*

In a small saucepan, bring the water to a boil. Remove from heat and add the herbs, cover, and steep for 30 minutes. Add the essential oil, stir, and strain.

Pour infusion into storage containers and shake well.

Refrigerate for up to 1 week, then discard.

APPLICATION TIPS: Using a cotton cleansing pad, apply approximately 1 teaspoon to the face or more as necessary for treating shoulder, back, or chest blemishes. Avoid eye area.

Herbal Astringent

This astringent thoroughly removes oil and perspiration without overdrying the skin. Use it following exercise, mowing the lawn, or doing anything that causes you to sweat profusely or get a bit greasy. It's perfect for someone who works in an oily, dirty, or greasy environment such as a commercial kitchen or garage.

1½   cups plain vodka (unsweetened and unflavored)

½   cup distilled water

1   teaspoon each sage, yarrow, chamomile flowers, rosemary, lemon balm, peppermint, and strawberry leaves

RECOMMENDED FOR: *oily, combination, acneic, or normal skin*
USE: *daily*
FOLLOW WITH: *moisturizer*
PREP TIME: *2 weeks, plus approximately 5 minutes to strain and bottle*
BLENDING TOOLS: *shake jar daily while steeping and before each use*
STORE IN: *plastic or glass bottle or spritzer*
YIELD: *approximately 2 cups*

Add all ingredients to a tightly lidded, pint-sized glass jar or canning jar and store in a dark, cool, dry cabinet to steep for 2 weeks, shaking the jar vigorously every day.

After this time, strain the liquid and pour into storage container(s).

No refrigeration is required, but for maximum freshness and potency, please use within 1 year.

APPLICATION TIPS: Using a cotton cleansing pad, apply approximately 1 teaspoon to the face or more as necessary to the shoulders or back. Avoid eye area.

Fresh Minty Astringent

This product is wonderful to use chilled in the warmer months. It has a cooling, fresh fragrance and can also be used as a men's aftershave or can be applied to women's legs, underarms, or bikini line (as tolerated; it will sting a bit) after shaving to prevent ingrown hairs.

2 tablespoons fresh, crushed peppermint, spearmint, or lemon balm (if dried, use 2 teaspoons of herb)	RECOMMENDED FOR: *oily, combination, acneic, or normal skin*
½ cup plain vodka (unsweetened and unflavored)	USE: *daily*
½ cup witch hazel	FOLLOW WITH: *moisturizer*

RECOMMENDED FOR: *oily, combination, acneic, or normal skin*
USE: *daily*
FOLLOW WITH: *moisturizer*
PREP TIME: *2 weeks, plus approximately 5 minutes to strain and bottle*
BLENDING TOOLS: *shake jar daily while steeping and before each use*
STORE IN: *plastic or glass bottle or spritzer*
YIELD: *approximately 1 cup*

Crush the fresh herb using a mortar and pestle. Combine the ingredients in a ½-pint or slightly larger jar with a tight-fitting lid. Allow the herb to steep for 2 weeks in a cool, dark, dry area, shaking vigorously every day.

After this time, strain the liquid and pour into a storage container.

No refrigeration is required, but for maximum freshness and potency, please use within 6 months.

APPLICATION TIPS: Using a cotton cleansing pad, apply approximately I teaspoon to the face or more as necessary to the shoulders or back. Avoid eye area.

SPICY AFTERSHAVE SKIN TONIC FOR MEN

*T*his tonic smells delightful, spicy, and masculine — but women like it, too! When strained, it can also be used as a scented hair rinse or scalp cleanser for oily or normal dark hair.

1   cup plain vodka (unsweetened and unflavored)
1   cup witch hazel
1   sprig fresh rosemary
1   sprig fresh mint of choice
1   cinnamon stick
5–10 whole cloves
2   strips fresh orange peel, cut into thin spirals
2   strips fresh lemon peel, cut into thin spirals
1   teaspoon vegetable glycerin
10 drops sweet orange essential oil
More citrus peels and spices (optional)

RECOMMENDED FOR: *all skin types except dry, dehydrated, sensitive, sunburned, windburned, or environmentally damaged skin*
USE: *daily*
FOLLOW WITH: *moisturizer*
PREP TIME: *2 weeks, plus approximately 10 minutes to strain and bottle*
BLENDING TOOLS: *shake jar daily while steeping and before each use*
STORE IN: *plastic or glass bottle or spritzer*
YIELD: *approximately 2 cups*

Combine all ingredients in a pint-size or slightly larger jar with a tight-fitting lid. Allow the mixture to steep for 2 weeks in a cool, dark, dry area, shaking vigorously every day.

After this time, strain the liquid and pour into storage container(s). You can add fresh citrus peels or spices to storage container(s) for aesthetic appeal (if desired).

No refrigeration is required, but for maximum freshness and potency, please use within 6 months.

APPLICATION TIPS: Using a cotton cleansing pad, apply approximately 1 teaspoon or use more as a facial splash after each shave.

Smooth-as-Velvet Vanilla Toner

*A*pply *this femininely fragranced toner right before a date when you want to smell sultry, soft, and sweet throughout the evening, or use it whenever you find your skin showing a bit of an oily sheen.*

1 cup plain vodka (unsweetened and unflavored)

1 cup distilled water

1 teaspoon vegetable glycerin

40 drops vanilla essential oil

RECOMMENDED FOR: *all skin types except very dry, sunburned, windburned, or dehydrated skin*
USE: *daily*
FOLLOW WITH: *moisturizer*
PREP TIME: *2 weeks, plus approximately 5 minutes to bottle*
BLENDING TOOLS: *shake jar daily while steeping and before each use*
STORE IN: *plastic or glass bottle or spritzer*
YIELD: *2 cups*

Combine all ingredients in a pint-size jar with a tight-fitting lid. Store in a cool, dark area for 2 weeks to steep, shaking vigorously every day.

After this time, pour into storage container(s).

No refrigeration is required, but for maximum freshness and potency, please use within 1 year.

APPLICATION TIPS: Using a cotton cleansing pad, apply approximately 1 teaspoon to the face or more as necessary to the shoulders or back. Avoid eye area.

OLD-FASHIONED LAVENDER TONER

The sweet, floral, relaxing aroma makes this a perfect toner for preteen girls.

1   tablespoon lavender buds

1   cup witch hazel

6   drops lavender essential oil

RECOMMENDED FOR: *oily, acneic, combination, or normal skin*
USE: *daily*
FOLLOW WITH: *moisturizer*
PREP TIME: *2 weeks, plus 5 minutes to strain and bottle*
BLENDING TOOLS: *shake jar daily while steeping and before each use*
STORE IN: *plastic or glass bottle or spritzer*
YIELD: *approximately 1 cup*

Combine ingredients in a tightly lidded, half-pint glass jar (or canning jar). Store in a cool, dark place for 2 weeks to steep, shaking vigorously every day.

After this time, strain the liquid and pour into storage container(s).

No refrigeration is required, but for maximum freshness and potency, please use within 6 months.

APPLICATION TIPS: Using a cotton cleansing pad, apply approximately 1 teaspoon to the face or more as necessary as a body splash. Avoid eye area.

HEALING HYDRATION TONIC

Comfrey and marsh mallow roots produce a very soothing mucilage that has wonderful healing and hydrating properties for all skin types. This tonic is excellent to use as a body splash in winter, when skin tends to be severely dry.

2	cups distilled water
1	heaping teaspoon comfrey root, chopped into small pieces
1	heaping teaspoon marsh mallow root, chopped into small pieces

RECOMMENDED FOR: *all skin types, especially dehydrated, sensitive, sunburned, windburned, mature, or environmentally damaged skin*
USE: *daily*
FOLLOW WITH: *moisturizer*
PREP TIME: *2 hours, plus approximately 5 to 10 minutes to strain and bottle*
BLENDING TOOLS: *shake before each use*
STORE IN: *plastic or glass bottle or spritzer*
YIELD: *approximately 2 cups*

In a small saucepan, bring the water to a boil, reduce heat to the lowest setting, add the herbs, cover, and steep for 1 hour. (Roots are tougher than leaves and flowers — thus a longer period of "cooking" is required to extract their healing components.) Then, turn off heat and remove pan to cool for 1 hour.

Pour the liquid through a strainer, mashing root bits as best you can with the back of a spoon to further extract the gooey, slippery mucilage.

Pour the liquid into storage container(s).

Refrigerate for up to 1 week, then discard.

APPLICATION TIPS: Using a cotton cleansing pad, apply approximately 1 teaspoon to the face or more as necessary for a body splash or wound wash. Avoid eye area.

FENNEL SOOTHER

This skin-softening product has a lovely, sweet, licorice-like fragrance and restores skin pH levels. It also softens hair if used as a hair rinse.

1 tablespoon crushed fennel seeds

2 cups distilled water

¼ cup raw apple cider vinegar

1 teaspoon vegetable glycerin

RECOMMENDED FOR: *all skin types, especially rashy or irritated skin*
USE: *daily*
FOLLOW WITH: *moisturizer*
PREP TIME: *45 minutes plus 5 minutes to strain and bottle*
BLENDING TOOLS: *mortar and pestle to crush seeds*
STORE IN: *plastic or glass bottle or spritzer*
YIELD: *approximately 2¼ cups*

Crush the seeds using a mortar and pestle. Boil the water, remove from heat, and add the crushed fennel seeds. Cover and allow the mixture to steep for 45 minutes. Add the vinegar and glycerin, then stir and strain the liquid.

Pour into storage container(s). Shake well to blend.

No refrigeration is required, but please use within 30 days, then discard.

APPLICATION TIPS: Using a cotton cleansing pad, apply approximately 1 teaspoon to the face or more as necessary for a body splash. Avoid eye area.

CHILLED CUCUMBER TONIC

*C*hilled cucumber juice is ever-so-soothing, calming, and hydrating. It's a classic for reducing swollen under eye "bags" and for helping skin recover from drying airplane travel.

1 medium cucumber, peeled, seeded, and cubed

2 tablespoons distilled or purified water

RECOMMENDED FOR: *all skin types, especially irritated, inflamed, dehydrated, sunburned, windburned, or itchy skin*
USE: *daily or when cucumbers are fresh and in season*
FOLLOW WITH: *moisturizer*
PREP TIME: *approximately 10 minutes*
BLENDING TOOLS: *blender*
STORE IN: *small plastic or glass jar*
YIELD: *varies; ¼ to ⅓ cup juice, depending on type and ripeness of cucumber*

Prepare the cucumber and place in a blender with water. Blend on medium or pulse if necessary until a thick, juicy pulp forms. Transfer the pulp into a strainer and catch the juice in a bowl.

Pour the juice into a storage container.

Refrigerate for up to 3 days, then discard.

APPLICATION TIPS: Using a cotton cleansing pad, apply approximately 1 teaspoon of juice to the face or more as necessary for other parts of the body. Avoid eye area.

ALOE VERA TONER

*A*loe vera juice makes a great all-over gentle toner. Contrary to popular belief, it's a bit drying if used routinely and is thus most effective for oily, combination, and normal skins in need of calming treatment and gentle handling. Aloe is extremely soothing and healing when used to relieve environmental irritations and the itch from insect bites. Note: Aloe vera may irritate very sensitive or dry, dehydrated, sunburned, or windburned skin. You can lessen the irritating effects and still benefit from its healing properties by diluting the juice or gel 50 percent with distilled water. Store the mixture in a small jar in the refrigerator and shake vigorously before each application.

Pure aloe vera juice or gel, commercially bottled or from fresh-picked leaf

RECOMMENDED FOR: *oily, acneic, combination, normal, or mature skin that is not dry; sunburned, windburned, or irritated skin*
USE: *daily*
FOLLOW WITH: *moisturizer*
PREP TIME: *none*
BLENDING TOOLS: *none*
STORE IN: *refrigerator in original container or store cut leaf in a plastic bag*
YIELD: *1 treatment*

If using commercial juice or gel, follow label directions regarding storage; it almost always requires refrigeration. If using the gel from a leaf of your own aloe plant, cut off the amount you are going to immediately need and store the remainder of the leaf in a plastic bag in the refrigerator. It will keep for about 3 days.

APPLICATION TIPS: Simply soak a cotton pad with the juice or gel and apply to skin as desired.

TANGERINE TONER

*T*his fragrant product that smells like the tropics can be made quickly and easily and is a good warm weather or "vacation" toner to keep on hand.

½ cup witch hazel
10 drops tangerine, neroli, or sweet orange essential oil

RECOMMENDED FOR: *all skin types except sensitive, dry, or dehydrated skin*
USE: *daily*
FOLLOW WITH: *moisturizer*
PREP TIME: *approximately 5 minutes*
BLENDING TOOLS: *shake before each use*
STORE IN: *plastic or glass bottle or spritzer*
YIELD: *½ cup*

Combine ingredients in a storage container and shake vigorously to blend.

No refrigeration is required, but for maximum freshness and potency, please use within 1 year.

APPLICATION TIPS: Using a cotton cleansing pad, apply approximately 1 teaspoon to the face or more as necessary to the shoulders, chest, or back. Avoid eye area.

ORANGE AND ROSE TONER

*T*his very gentle and soothing toner softens and moisturizes chapped, weather-beaten skin.

1   cup distilled water
1   tablespoon crumbled,
    dried orange rind
1   teaspoon rose petals
1   tablespoon vegetable
    glycerin

RECOMMENDED FOR: *combination, normal, dry, mature, sunburned or windburned, sensitive, or environmentally damaged skin*
USE: *daily*
FOLLOW WITH: *moisturizer*
PREP TIME: *45 minutes plus 5 minutes to strain and bottle*
BLENDING TOOLS: *shake before each use*
STORE IN: *plastic or glass bottle or spritzer*
YIELD: *approximately 1 cup*

In a small saucepan, bring the water to a boil, remove from heat, add the herbs, cover, and steep for 45 minutes. Strain into a storage container and add the glycerin. Shake vigorously to blend.

Refrigerate for up to 1 week, then discard.

APPLICATION TIPS: Using a cotton cleansing pad, apply approximately 1 teaspoon to the face or more as necessary to the body. Avoid eye area.

ELDER FLOWER TONER

*T*his healing, calming, and ever-so-gentle tonic can even be used to soothe the skin of an infant suffering from dermatitis or eczema.

1   cup distilled water
1   tablespoon elder flowers
1   tablespoon vegetable glycerin
5   drops lavender essential oil (optional)

RECOMMENDED FOR: *all skin types, especially sensitive, dry, dehydrated, sunburned or windburned, mature, or environmentally damaged skin*
USE: *daily*
FOLLOW WITH: *moisturizer*
PREP TIME: *45 minutes plus 5 minutes to strain and bottle*
BLENDING TOOLS: *shake before each use*
STORE IN: *plastic or glass bottle or spritzer*
YIELD: *approximately 1 cup*

In a small saucepan, bring the water to a boil, remove from heat, add the herb, cover, and steep for 45 minutes. Strain and pour into a storage container. Add the glycerin and the essential oil (if desired). Shake vigorously to blend.

Refrigerate for up to 1 week, then discard.

APPLICATION TIPS: Using a cotton cleansing pad, apply approximately 1 teaspoon to the face or more as necessary to the body. Avoid eye area.

Tea Tree and Thyme Healing Tonic

*T*his recipe makes a very strong infusion of thyme. Combined with tea tree, the resultant formula has antiseptic, antibacterial, antifungal, and antiviral properties and makes a good preventive skin tonic to use when living or working around people who have a cold or the flu. Pour it into a small, plastic spritzer bottle and keep it with you at all times so that you can spray it periodically on your hands and face, the telephone, and directly into the air to help purify the surrounding environment.

1 cup distilled water
1 tablespoon
   thyme leaves
10 drops tea tree essential oil

RECOMMENDED FOR: *all skin types, especially those with weeping acne, abrasions, burns, infections, inflamed eczema, or psoriasis*
USE: *daily or as needed*
FOLLOW WITH: *moisturizer*
PREP TIME: *approximately 35 minutes, plus 5 minutes to strain and bottle*
BLENDING TOOLS: *shake before each use*
STORE IN: *plastic or glass bottle or spritzer*
YIELD: *approximately 1 cup*

In a small saucepan, bring the water to a boil, remove from heat, add the herb, cover, and steep for 30 minutes. Strain and pour the liquid into a storage container. Add the essential oil. Shake vigorously to blend.

Due to tea tree essential oil's potent properties, this tonic will keep unrefrigerated for approximately 1 week. Please make a fresh batch every weekend so you're prepared to naturally combat the upcoming week's exposure to germs!

APPLICATION TIPS: Using a cotton cleansing pad, apply approximately 1 teaspoon to the face or more as necessary for other parts of the body. Avoid eye area.

Masks

The use of masks for the beautification and purification of both the face and body dates back to ancient civilizations. Clay was especially valued for its color variations; its ability to absorb animal, mineral, and botanical dyes; and its use as body paint during important rituals and events.

Today, though, masks are used primarily for cosmetic purposes to deep-clean the skin. Depending on their ingredients, they can increase circulation, remove toxins, tone and tighten, act as nonabrasive exfoliants, hydrate and moisturize, calm inflammation, and soften the skin. Masks can be made from myriad natural ingredients such as various clays, brewer's yeast, or grains, which absorb excess oil and dead cells from the skin's surface and stimulate a sluggish complexion. Masks can also be made from such succulent ingredients as fresh, ripe peaches and cream, which moisturize and bring a glow to a dry complexion.

PREPARATION TIP: Because recipes are mixed for a single use, purified water may be used in lieu of distilled water.

APPLICATION TIPS: Be sure to pull your hair off your face and neck — some of the juicier masks have a habit of trickling down a bit into places where they're not welcome. A mask should always be applied to freshly cleansed, barely damp skin. For specific application tips and times, see individual recipes.

Everyone's Basic Clay Mask

All clay masks gently exfoliate as they tighten, stimulate circulation, remineral-ize, and soften the skin. Because it can be customized according to skin type, this mask is gentle enough to be used by anyone. If mixed with water, it makes an excellent overnight pimple treatment. Simply apply a dab to each pimple with a cotton swab and leave on while you sleep. In the morning, rinse off the remaining bits of mask with warm water. The clay absorbs excess oil during the night and aids in the healing of blemishes.

1 tablespoon white clay
Cream (for dry skin),
  milk (low fat or whole;
  for normal skin), or
  water (for oily skin)

RECOMMENDED FOR: *all skin types*
USE: *1 or 2 times per week*
FOLLOW WITH: *moisturizer*
PREP TIME: *approximately 5 minutes*
BLENDING TOOLS: *small bowl, spoon or tiny whisk*
STORE IN: *do not store; mix as needed*
YIELD: *1 treatment*

In a small bowl, combine the clay with enough of the appropriate liquid (determined by your skin type) to form a smooth, spreadable paste. Give it a few stirs with a small spoon or tiny whisk to remove any lumps.

APPLICATION TIPS: Using fingers, spread paste onto the face, neck, and décolleté (if desired), and allow to dry completely for 20 to 30 minutes, preferably while you are lying down. The mask will seemingly lift and tighten the skin. Rinse.

GREEN GODDESS PURIFYING CLAY MASK

You can also apply this drying mask to chest or back areas that have blemishes. French green clay combined with either of the highly anti-inflammatory essential oils is very healing for sensitive, cystic, and weeping acne conditions: It aids in removing impurities and toxins from beneath the surface of the skin. This mask is the preferred method of exfoliation for acneic skin due to its gentleness. (Most granular, chemical, enzyme, and fruit acid masks can be quite irritating to acneic skin.) It can also serve as an overnight blemish treatment. Simply apply a dab on each pimple with a cotton swab and leave on while you sleep. In the morning, rinse off the remaining bits of mask with warm water. The clay absorbs excess oil during the night and aids in the healing of blemishes.

1 tablespoon French green clay, finely ground

Pure aloe vera juice

2 drops German chamomile or helichrysum essential oil

RECOMMENDED FOR: *oily, acneic, combination, or oily mature skin*
USE: *1 or 2 times per week*
FOLLOW WITH: *moisturizer*
PREP TIME: *approximately 5 minutes*
BLENDING TOOLS: *small bowl and spoon or tiny whisk*
STORE IN: *do not store; mix as needed*
YIELD: *1 treatment*

In a small bowl, use a spoon or whisk to combine the clay with enough of the aloe vera juice to form a smooth, spreadable paste. Stir in the essential oil.

APPLICATION TIPS: Using fingers, spread paste onto the face and neck and allow to dry completely for 20 to 30 minutes, preferably while you are lying down. The mask will seemingly lift and tighten the skin. Rinse.

Egg White Firming Mask

This mask can dramatically tone your skin and visibly shrink your pores. Its results are amazing, if only temporary. You'll swear you've had a mini-face-lift when you're finished! Note: *Be aware that egg whites and cornstarch form a very tightening duo; this combination will leave you unable to comfortably move your mouth when it completely dries.*

White of 1 cold, fresh small
    or medium egg

1   teaspoon cornstarch

RECOMMENDED FOR: *all skin types, especially skin with large pores and slack, saggy tone*
USE: *1 or 2 times per week or as desired*
FOLLOW WITH: *moisturizer*
PREP TIME: *5 to 10 minutes*
BLENDING TOOLS: *small bowl and fork or small whisk*
STORE IN: *do not store; mix as needed*
YIELD: *1 treatment*

Combine the egg white and cornstarch in a small bowl or drinking glass and beat with a fork or small whisk until foamy and well blended. The mixture should not be lumpy.

APPLICATION TIPS: Using fingers, smooth the gooey, gel-like mask onto the face and throat in a thin, even coat. You must lie down while this dries or gravity will pull your face and any wrinkles you have downward — which is not what you want! If you have a slanted chaise or a board that you can arrange in a slant, lie on this while your mask is drying for approximately 20 minutes. Rinse.

Rosy Red Balancing Clay Mask

*T*his mask is wonderfully fragrant, tightening, lifting, mineralizing, and sebum-balancing. It can also serve as an excellent overnight blemish treatment. Simply apply a dab on each pimple with a cotton swab and leave on while you sleep. In the morning, rinse off the remaining bits of mask with warm water. The clay absorbs excess oil during the night and aids in the healing of blemishes.

1   tablespoon red clay, finely ground

Rose, rose geranium, or neroli hydrosol

2   drops rose otto, geranium, or neroli essential oil

RECOMMENDED FOR: *oily, acneic, combination, normal, or oily-to-normal mature skin*
USE: *1 or 2 times per week*
FOLLOW WITH: *moisturizer*
PREP TIME: *approximately 5 minutes*
BLENDING TOOLS: *small bowl and spoon or whisk*
STORE IN: *plastic or glass jar, zip-seal bag, or tin (dry ingredient only)*
YIELD: *1 treatment*

In a small bowl, use a spoon or whisk to combine the clay with enough of the hydrosol of choice to form a smooth, spreadable paste. Stir in the essential oil.

APPLICATION TIPS: Using fingers, spread paste onto the face and neck and allow to dry completely for 20 to 30 minutes, preferably while you are lying down. The clay will seemingly lift and tighten the skin. Rinse.

YOGURT EXFOLIATING AND BLEACHING MASK

Yogurt is great for a fading tan or for blotchy, uneven skin. With repeated use, it slightly bleaches and evens skin tone. Plain yogurt is also a very gentle, soothing, nonabrasive exfoliant that becomes more effective with repeated use.

1 tablespoon plain yogurt

RECOMMENDED FOR: *all skin types except very sensitive skin*
USE: *1 to 2 times per week or as desired*
FOLLOW WITH: *moisturizer*
PREP TIME: *approximately 1 minute*
BLENDING TOOLS: *small spoon*
STORE IN: *original container in the refrigerator*
YIELD: *1 treatment*

APPLICATION TIPS: Using fingers or a cosmetic fan brush, apply yogurt to the face, neck, and décolleté. Be sure to lie down; the yogurt can become a bit runny when it reaches skin temperature. Leave on for 20 to 30 minutes. Even though the mask may not be completely dry, rinse.

BREWER'S YEAST MASK

This mask stimulates circulation and delivers a definite rosy glow, making it perfect for the sluggish or clogged complexion. It may tingle as it dries and quickly tightens the skin — but this is normal. If it starts to sting beyond your comfort level, rinse it off immediately with cool water and apply a good moisturizer.

1 tablespoon edible brewer's yeast flakes	RECOMMENDED FOR: *oily, combination, acneic, normal, or oily mature skin*
2 teaspoons milk (nonfat or low fat) or water	USE: *1 to 2 times per week*
	FOLLOW WITH: *moisturizer*
	PREP TIME: *approximately 5 minutes*
	BLENDING TOOLS: *small bowl and spoon*
	STORE IN: *do not store; mix as needed*
	YIELD: *1 treatment*

Combine ingredients in a small bowl to form a smooth paste. You may need more or less liquid than called for, depending on the brand of yeast used and the size of the flakes.

APPLICATION TIPS: Using fingers, spread onto the face and throat in a thin layer. If the chest or back is blemished, make additional amounts and apply there as well. When the mask has dried in approximately 20 minutes, rinse with cool water to calm skin.

Papaya No-More-Pores Double Mask Treatment

This mask's slight bleaching action helps even skin tone and leaves skin with a wonderful glow. The papaya and pineapple contain protein-dissolving enzymes (papain and bromelain, respectively) that help to dissolve and lift away dry scaly skin, which, over time, can build up on your skin and leave a dull appearance. With repeated use, this mask will tend to make your pores appear smaller (likely due to the removal of dead skin debris, which can clog and stretch the pore wall).

Mask 1

¼ cup freshly mashed raw papaya

1 teaspoon fresh, raw pineapple juice (optional)

RECOMMENDED FOR: *all skin types except sensitive, irritated, sunburned, or windburned skin; use as tolerated on environmentally damaged skin*
USE: *1 time per week*
FOLLOW WITH: *moisturizer*
PREP TIME: *10 to 15 minutes*
BLENDING TOOLS: *mortar and pestle or small bowl and fork*
STORE IN: *do not store; mix as needed*
YIELD: *1 treatment for Mask 1; 1 treatment for Mask 2*

Using a mortar and pestle or a small bowl and fork, mash the papaya and combine with the pineapple juice (if available and desired) until the two are thoroughly mixed and a smooth paste is formed.

APPLICATION TIPS: Gently pat this juicy pulp onto the face and neck with your fingers, then lie down for 15 to 20 minutes with a towel around your head and behind your neck — the product can be a bit runny. Your face will probably tingle during this time but you can relax; it just means the natural fruit acids are working. After 20 minutes, rinse.

Mask 2

After using the papaya Mask 1, apply Everyone's Basic Clay Mask (page 146), using strong sage or rosemary tea or an infusion made with 1 teaspoon of herb (see page 59, How to Make an Herbal Infusion) in place of the cream, milk, or water as the liquid to mix with the clay. *Note:* If your skin is especially sensitive or irritated, use milk or cream as the mixing liquid.

APPLICATION TIPS: Apply as directed in the recipe. Those with dry skin can apply a thin layer of moisturizer before proceeding with the clay mask. All skin types should apply moisturizer *after* this mask. After you've finished, your face will look smoother and more refined.

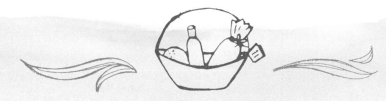

Mask Gift Idea

Several mask recipes offered here can be packaged and given as gifts. These include masks based on dry ingredients such as clay, ground oatmeal, sunflower seed meal, brewer's yeast, and almond meal.

- Prepare a few batches of these base ingredients and divide ½-cup measurements into individual plastic bags that can be tightly sealed.
- With ribbon or twine, attach to the bag instructions for preparing and using the mask.
- Place several bags in a decorative tin or small wooden box and decorate the exterior with a personalized label.

Honey and Wheat Germ Softening Mask

*H*oney acts as a humectant, drawing moisture from the air to the skin, thus this mask is deeply soothing, moisturizing, and hydrating. It's wonderful to use during the cold, dry winter season or if you live in an area with low humidity and is perfect if you do a great deal of traveling via airplane.

1   tablespoon fresh, raw honey
1   teaspoon sunflower seed meal
1   teaspoon fresh, raw wheat germ

RECOMMENDED FOR: *all skin types, especially dry, dehydrated, sensitive and environmentally damaged skin*
USE: *as often as desired*
FOLLOW WITH: *moisturizer if necessary*
PREP TIME: *approximately 5 minutes*
BLENDING TOOLS: *small bowl and spoon*
STORE IN: *do not store; mix as needed*
YIELD: *1 treatment*

Thoroughly combine all ingredients in a small bowl and allow to set for a couple of minutes.

APPLICATION TIPS: Pat onto the face and neck with your fingers, then lie down, relax, and leave on for approximately 30 minutes. After the allotted time, rinse with a very warm, damp cloth. The honey will become thinner and have a tendency to run as it warms to body temperature, so be sure to tuck your hair away from your face prior to application or you'll have a sticky mess. You may want to place a towel behind your head as well.

DEEP PORE CLEANSER

This recipe is quite soothing and has a slight astringent and bleaching action. The product doubles as a facial scrub.

¼ medium-sized ripe, peeled, seeded, chopped tomato or 2-inch chunk of cucumber, peeled, seeded and chopped

Water

1 teaspoon almond meal

1 teaspoon ground oatmeal

1 teaspoon sunflower seed meal

¼ teaspoon favorite base oil, such as almond, apricot kernel, hazelnut, jojoba, or extra-virgin olive

RECOMMENDED FOR: *oily, combination, normal, or oily mature skin*
USE: *1 to 2 times per week*
FOLLOW WITH: *moisturizer*
PREP TIME: *10 to 15 minutes (if meals are ground ahead of time)*
BLENDING TOOLS: *blender, small bowl and spoon*
STORE IN: *do not store; mix as needed*
YIELD: *1 treatment*

Place tomato or cucumber in a blender and add a small amount of water (one tablespoon at most). Blend until smooth.

Strain this vegetable liquid and, in a small bowl, combine enough of the liquid with the meals and base oil to form a smooth, spreadable paste.

APPLICATION TIPS: Using your fingers, spread paste onto the face and neck as thickly as possible and allow it to remain on skin for 20 minutes. Even if the mask isn't dry after this time, rinse skin.

PEACHES AND CREAM GLOW MASK

*T*his mask is as aromatic and delicious as it is nourishing and moisturizing for your skin. I have included enough of the ingredients so that you can eat a spoonful or two of the mixture before putting it on your skin. You may even be tempted to mix up a larger batch, add a dab of honey, and drink it for lunch! The flavor and smell of this mask is reminiscent of real homemade peach ice cream — summery, sweet, and smooth.

½ very ripe, small peach, peeled, or ¼ medium peach

1 tablespoon heavy cream

RECOMMENDED FOR: *normal, dry, dehydrated, sensitive, mature, or environmentally damaged skin*
USE: *as desired*
FOLLOW WITH: *moisturizer if necessary*
PREP TIME: *approximately 5 minutes*
BLENDING TOOLS: *mortar and pestle or small bowl and fork*
STORE IN: *do not store; mix as needed*
YIELD: *1 treatment*

Using a mortar and pestle or a small bowl and fork, mash the peach and combine with the cream until smooth.

APPLICATION TIPS: Using your fingers, apply mixture to the face, neck, and décolleté (if desired), and leave on for 30 minutes while lying down or reclining with feet elevated. If you have a slanted chaise or a board that you can arrange in a slant, lie on this while your mask is drying. It's a bit runny, so wear the necessary hair and protective towels to catch any drips. After the allotted time, rinse.

APPLESAUCE AND WHEAT GERM MOISTURIZING MASK

This treatment leaves skin ultra-moisturized and is soothing to use (especially if the product is chilled) on hot, sunburned, or windburned skin.

2	teaspoons fresh applesauce
2	teaspoons raw wheat germ
½	teaspoon jojoba, hazelnut, apricot kernel, or almond base oil

RECOMMENDED FOR: *normal, dry, mature, sensitive, environmentally damaged, sunburned, or windburned skin*
USE: *as desired*
FOLLOW WITH: *moisturizer if necessary*
PREP TIME: *approximately 10 minutes*
BLENDING TOOLS: *small bowl and spoon*
STORE IN: *do not store; mix as needed*
YIELD: *1 treatment*

In a small bowl, thoroughly mix the applesauce and wheat germ. Allow the mixture to thicken for 5 minutes or until the wheat germ absorbs some of the apple juice. Have the oil ready to use after the mask application.

APPLICATION TIPS: Using your fingers, apply to the face, neck, and décolleté (if desired). This is another mask that can be a bit messy; wrap up your hair, take a load off your feet, lie back, and think pleasant thoughts while your skin drinks in all this nourishing moisture. Rinse after 20 or 30 minutes, even though the mask may not be dry.

Follow with a nourishing oil facial massage: For 5 minutes, simply massage the chosen base oil into your face, neck, and décolleté using gentle, circular motions. Remove any excess oil by gently patting your skin with a tissue or massage the residual oil into your arms, knees, feet, or any part in need of softening. Your face will be moist, warm, and glowing.

Honey Massage Mask

This is a delicious, sweet way to soften, deeply hydrate, and moisturize your skin. This treatment leaves skin with a rosy glow resulting from increased circulation.

2–3 teaspoons fresh, raw honey at room temperature

RECOMMENDED FOR: *all skin types, especially dry, dehydrated, sunburned, windburned, mature, or environmentally damaged skin*
USE: *as desired*
FOLLOW WITH: *moisturizer if necessary*
PREP TIME: *approximately 1 minute*
BLENDING TOOLS: *small spoon*
STORE IN: *do not store; mix as needed*
YIELD: *1 treatment*

APPLICATION TIPS: Honey thins and gets runnier as it warms to skin temperature, so be sure to wear a shower cap or pull your hair off your face and neck prior to application. Using your fingers, apply a very thin coat of honey to your entire face, neck, and décolleté. When the honey is spread evenly, it will bead on your skin much like water beads on your car after a rain shower. Leave on for 15 minutes or longer while you lie down and rest. Your skin will begin to feel very warm and relaxed. Don't fall asleep! Before rinsing, for about 5 minutes, begin to pat your skin lightly with your fingertips in quick tapping motions, as though you are playing the piano. Rinse using a very warm, damp cloth.

Avocado and Buttermilk Mask

*T*his incredibly nourishing and moisturizing mask with slight bleaching action leaves skin feeling velvety soft. Make a larger batch to apply to hair; it serves as an effective conditioning treatment for normal, dry, and chemically damaged or frizzy hair. After applying to hair, cover your head with plastic wrap or a shower cap and leave on for 30 minutes. Rinse and shampoo.

¼ very ripe, small avocado
Buttermilk

RECOMMENDED FOR: *normal to very dry and mature skin, especially rough, dehydrated, chapped, or environmentally damaged skin*
USE: *as desired*
FOLLOW WITH: *moisturizer if necessary*
PREP TIME: *approximately 5 minutes*
BLENDING TOOLS: *mortar and pestle or small bowl and fork*
STORE IN: *do not store; mix as needed*
YIELD: *1 treatment*

Scoop out the avocado pulp and mash it with just enough buttermilk to form a creamy paste. A mortar and pestle or small bowl and fork work equally well for this.

APPLICATION TIPS: This mask can be a bit runny, so safeguard your hair and clothes prior to application. Using your fingers, apply paste in upward strokes to the face, neck, and décolleté. If possible, use in the early morning and lie in the early sun to allow the oils of the avocado to warm and penetrate your skin. Rinse after 20 to 30 minutes.

Oatmeal Mask

This mask acts as a gentle exfoliant. Its slight bleaching action helps even blotchy skin tone if used at least twice per week.

4   teaspoons ground
    oatmeal
5   teaspoons buttermilk

RECOMMENDED FOR: *all skin types except very sensitive, sunburned, windburned, or irritated skin*
USE: *as desired*
FOLLOW WITH: *moisturizer*
PREP TIME: *approximately 5 minutes (if oatmeal is ground ahead of time)*
BLENDING TOOLS: *small bowl and spoon*
STORE IN: *do not store; mix as needed*
YIELD: *1 treatment*

In a small bowl, combine both ingredients. Allow the mixture to thicken for a few minutes, then give it a few stirs again to remove any lumps. If it's too thick, add a tad more buttermilk; if it's too thin, add more ground oats.

APPLICATION TIPS: Using your fingers, spread onto the face, throat, and décolleté. If you have a slanted chaise or a board that you can arrange in a slant, lie down with your head lower than your feet while your mask is drying for 20 to 30 minutes. Rinse.

GREEN ALGAE NOURISHMENT MASK

Algae is an aquatic plant that is chock-full of valuable vitamin A and trace miner-als. As stated in chapter 1, it's equally as nourishing to consume as it is to apply to your skin.

1 tablespoon powdered
   green algae (any variety)
Pure aloe vera juice

RECOMMENDED FOR: *oily, combination, normal, or oily mature skin*
USE: *1 or 2 times per week*
FOLLOW WITH: *moisturizer*
PREP TIME: *approximately 5 minutes*
BLENDING TOOLS: *small bowl and spoon*
STORE IN: *do not store; mix as needed*
YIELD: *1 treatment*

In a small bowl, combine the algae with just enough aloe vera juice to form a spreadable paste. Allow the mixture to thicken for about 1 minute.

APPLICATION TIPS: Using your fingers, spread onto the face and throat, lie back, and let the mask dry for 20 to 30 minutes. Rinse.

Mellow Yellow Banana Cream Mask

Bananas and cream will moisturize, hydrate, and pamper even the driest skin. Try to make this mask a healthy, yummy habit that your skin will relish. Note: Should a bit of this delectably scrumptious mask drip into your mouth, it's fine to savor it!

I   2-inch chunk of a
     very ripe banana
Cream, light or heavy

RECOMMENDED FOR: *normal, dry, dehydrated, sensitive, sunburned, windburned, environmentally damaged, mature, or irritated skin*
USE: *as desired*
FOLLOW WITH: *moisturizer if necessary*
PREP TIME: *approximately 5 minutes*
BLENDING TOOLS: *mortar and pestle or small bowl and fork*
STORE IN: *do not store; mix as needed*
YIELD: *1 treatment*

Using a mortar and pestle or a small bowl and fork, mash the banana with just enough cream until a smooth, spreadable paste forms.

APPLICATION TIPS: Safeguard hair and clothing prior to applying this potentially runny mask. Using your fingers, spread onto the face, throat, and décolleté, and recline for 20 to 30 minutes (mask will not dry). Rinse.

Vanilla and Cream Firming Mask

This is a delicately fragranced mask that tightens and moisturizes and leaves skin clarified and smooth. It can be used by those with even the most sensitive and dry skin.

1 tablespoon white clay, finely ground

Cream, light or heavy

2 drops vanilla essential oil

RECOMMENDED FOR: *all skin types*
USE: *1 or 2 times per week*
FOLLOW WITH: *moisturizer if necessary*
PREP TIME: *approximately 5 minutes*
BLENDING TOOLS: *small bowl and spoon*
STORE IN: *do not store; mix as needed*
YIELD: *1 treatment*

In a small bowl, combine the clay with just enough cream to form a spreadable paste. Stir in the essential oil.

APPLICATION TIPS: Using your fingers, spread onto the face and throat, then lie down and relax for 20 to 30 minutes until the mask dries. Rinse.

Raspberry Refining Mask

This mask gently exfoliates, tightens, and bleaches dull, slack, blotchy skin, leaving behind a "raspberry" radiance. Note: Though it smells yummy, don't eat this one — the clay makes it gritty!

¼ cup fresh raspberries, or thawed if purchased frozen

Purified water (if berries are dry)

2 teaspoons white clay, finely ground

2 teaspoons ground oatmeal

RECOMMENDED FOR: *all skin types except dry, dehydrated, sensitive, sunburned, or windburned skin; use as tolerated on environmentally damaged skin*
USE: *1 or 2 times per week*
FOLLOW WITH: *moisturizer*
PREP TIME: *approximately 10 minutes (if oatmeal is ground ahead of time)*
BLENDING TOOLS: *mortar and pestle or small bowl and fork*
STORE IN: *do not store; mix as needed*
YIELD: *1 treatment*

Using a mortar and pestle or a small bowl and fork, mash the raspberries until nearly smooth. This should produce a runny pulp. Don't worry about the seeds; they should be included. If the berries are on the dry side, add a little water until the pulp is quite juicy. Stir in the clay and oats until a spreadable paste forms. Allow the oats and clay to absorb moisture and thicken for a minute or two. If the resulting mixture is too thick, add more water; if it's too thin, add more oats.

APPLICATION TIPS: Using your fingers, spread paste onto the face, throat, and décolleté (if desired), then lie down and rest while the mask dries. If it happens to be runny, safeguard hair and clothing prior to application. Rinse after 20 to 30 minutes, even if the mask isn't dry.

Herbal Facial Steams

An herbal facial steam has an almost magical ability to transform a dreary, sluggish, parched, lackluster complexion into a dewy, glowing, supple, younger version of itself. Warm, moist heat encourages the pores to perspire and breathe. It also imparts vital moisture to deeper skin layers, relaxes muscle tissue, plumps wrinkles, boosts circulation, and brings oxygenated blood to the surface of skin. Finally, steam coaxes the facial tissues to relinquish toxins. As the steam penetrates the skin, the various herbs release their volatile oils and act as astringents or tonics to aid in healing. Any clogging from sebum, dirt, or makeup is dislodged for easy removal, thus causing pores to appear less prominent.

CONTRAINDICATIONS: Herbal steams may be used regularly by all skin types with the exception of acneic skin with weepy active or cystic acne or acne, rosacea; sensitive, sunburned, or windburned skin; or skin with broken capillaries. Heat can further irritate these conditions.

PREPARATION TIPS: To prepare for a facial steam, first thoroughly cleanse your skin. Next, boil 3 cups distilled or purified water. If a recipe calls for vinegar, boil it with the water. Remove the liquid from heat and add the herbs, cover, and steep for 5 minutes. Then add any other ingredients listed in the recipe, such as base oil or essential oils.

APPLICATION TIPS: Place the pot of infused herbs in a stable place where you can sit comfortably for 10 minutes. Remove the cover from the pan, drape a large bath towel over your head, shoulders, and the steaming herb pot to create a tent. With your eyes closed and your face 10 to 12 inches from the edge of the pot (to avoid burning your skin), breathe deeply and relax. Keep your eyes closed during the entire steam. When finished, splash your face and neck with tepid water, followed by a few splashes of cool water. Pat skin until almost dry. For a full facial treatment, finish by using a mask and moisturizer.

Note: If you'd like to make a larger batch of your favorite facial steam mixture to have handy for yourself or gift-giving, store the dry ingredients in an air-tight zip-seal bag, plastic or glass jar, or tin, and keep it in a cool, dark place for 6 to 12 months. Add the water and oil or vinegar whenever you're ready for a facial steam.

What can you do with the leftover herbal liquid after you've steamed your face? If it doesn't contain vinegar, let it cool, strain it, and use it to water your plants, add it to your bath water, or pour the whole mixture onto your compost pile. It needn't go to waste!

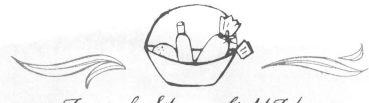

Facial Steam Gift Idea

An attractive container for facial steam ingredients is a 2 quart-size, old-fashioned speckled enameled pot.

- Make about ½ cup of the herb mixture from one of the following recipes.
- Put it in a plastic freezer bag and tie the bag closed with a ribbon or twine.
- Attach mixing instructions and a measuring spoon.
- Place the bag inside the pot (which can be used to make the facial steam). A nice accompaniment is a bath towel. If you can, choose a towel and pot that are the same color.

BASIC STEAM

This mixture contains soothing, healing, and slightly astringent herbs to help balance and tighten all skin types. It can double as a stimulating hair rinse for light brown and blonde/red hair.

3   cups distilled water
1   teaspoon calendula blossoms
1   teaspoon chamomile flowers
2   teaspoons raspberry, blackberry, or strawberry leaves
1   teaspoon peppermint (optional)

RECOMMENDED FOR: *all skin types (except those types listed in Contraindications on page 165)*
USE: *1 or 2 times per week*
FOLLOW WITH: *moisturizer*
PREP TIME: *approximately 15 minutes*
STORE IN: *do not store; mix as needed*
YIELD: *1 treatment*

PREPARATION AND APPLICATION TIPS: Follow general directions on page 165.

To use as a hair rinse, strain, cool, and pour entire recipe over hair after conditioning.

REFRESHING PORE CLEANSER

All the herbs in this mix have the ability to tighten the skin, combat excessive oili-ness, and stimulate circulation.

3   cups distilled water
1   teaspoon yarrow
1   teaspoon sage
1   teaspoon rosemary
1   teaspoon peppermint

RECOMMENDED FOR: *oily, combination, normal, or oily mature skin (except those types listed in Contraindications on page 165)*
USE: *1 or 2 times per week*
FOLLOW WITH: *moisturizer*
PREP TIME: *approximately 15 minutes*
STORE IN: *do not store; mix as needed*
YIELD: *1 treatment*

PREPARATION AND APPLICATION TIPS: Follow general directions on page 165.

Steam pH Balancer

This facial steam is particularly effective if you wear foundation makeup daily or use soap to cleanse your skin — both can leave behind a drying, alkaline film, resulting in patchy dryness, dull skin, and clogged pores. Your skin is naturally a bit on the acid side with a pH of approximately 5 to 6. The vinegar in this steam helps restore your skin's proper pH balance and leaves skin feeling very fresh and soft.

3	cups distilled water
¼	cup apple cider vinegar
1	teaspoon lavender buds
1	teaspoon rosemary
1	teaspoon rose petals

RECOMMENDED FOR: *all skin types (except those types listed in Contraindications on page 165)*
USE: *1 or 2 times per week*
FOLLOW WITH: *moisturizer*
PREP TIME: *approximately 15 minutes*
STORE IN: *do not store; mix as needed*
YIELD: *1 treatment*

PREPARATION AND APPLICATION TIPS: Follow general directions on page 165.

Please keep eyes closed while taking this steam; the vinegar may sting or cause excessive training.

Dry Skin Sauna

This steam is like a gentle spring rain for your skin: pampering and hydrating. It doubles as a toner.

3   cups distilled water
1   teaspoon calendula blossoms
1   teaspoon comfrey leaves
1   teaspoon elder flowers
1   teaspoon favorite base oil

RECOMMENDED FOR: *normal, dry, mature, environmentally damaged, and sensitive skin (except those types listed in Contraindications on page 165)*
USE: *1 to 2 times per week*
FOLLOW WITH: *moisturizer*
PREP TIME: *approximately 15 minutes*
STORE IN: *plastic or glass bottle (if using as a toner) — otherwise, do not store; mix as needed*
YIELD: *1 treatment*

PREPARATION AND APPLICATION TIPS: Follow general directions on page 165.

TO USE AS A TONER: Strain, cool, and bottle, and store in refrigerator for up to 1 week. Shake before each use.

WRINKLE CHASER

If you like the scent of licorice and roses, you'll love this steam and its hydrating, wrinkle-relaxing effects on your skin. The sweet aroma is mildly stimulating yet balancing to the psyche.

3 cups distilled water

1 tablespoon fennel seeds, crushed

2 drops rose otto or geranium essential oil

RECOMMENDED FOR: *all skin types, especially dehydrated, environmentally damaged, mature, rough, and chapped (except those types listed in Contraindications on page 165)*

USE: *1 or 2 times per week*
FOLLOW WITH: *moisturizer*
PREP TIME: *approximately 15 minutes*
BLENDING TOOLS: *mortar and pestle*
STORE IN: *do not store; mix as needed*
YIELD: *1 treatment*

PREPARATION AND APPLICATION TIPS: Follow general directions on page 165, adding the crushed seeds to the boiling water.

Aromatherapeutic Express Facial Steams

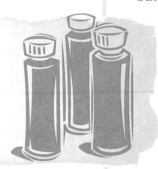

The following recipes don't require blending and brewing herbs, but simply call for the use of highly therapeutic essential oils — meaning express steams takes less time to prepare than the previous steam recipes here. No steeping needed!

Essential oils are concentrated and have varied properties. In taking these steams, your entire being will reap a wealth of healing goodness.

ROSE GERANIUM AND LAVENDER EXPRESS STEAM

*B*oth lavender and geranium oils have balancing properties with regard to sebum production in the skin. The aroma of this steam helps reduce stress, anxiety, and fatigue.

3	cups distilled water
3	drops geranium essential oil
3	drops lavender essential oil

RECOMMENDED FOR: *all skin types (except those types listed in Contraindications on page 165)*
USE: *1 or 2 times per week*
FOLLOW WITH: *moisturizer*
PREP TIME: *approximately 5 minutes*
STORE IN: *do not store; mix as needed*
YIELD: *1 treatment*

PREPARATION AND APPLICATION TIPS: Follow general directions on page 165.

CONGESTION RELIEF EXPRESS STEAM

This steam not only helps clear congested or blemished, clogged, oily skin, but also aids in relieving sinus and lung congestion and sinus headache due to allergy, flu, or cold symptoms. I swear by this steam when I have a bad head cold or when my lungs feel heavy and oxygen flow is diminished. It really helps drain away the misery and seems to open up everything! A bonus: The stimulating aroma also leaves your house smelling cool and clean.

3   cups distilled water
2   drops **each** of the following essential oils: peppermint; eucalyptus (*E. radiata*); juniper; ravensara

RECOMMENDED FOR: *all skin types' especially oily, combination, normal, or oily mature skin (except for those types listed in Contraindications on page 165)*
USE: *1 or 2 times per week*
FOLLOW WITH: *moisturizer*
PREP TIME: *approximately 5 minutes*
STORE IN: *do not store; mix as needed*
YIELD: *1 treatment*

PREPARATION AND APPLICATION TIPS: Follow general directions on page 165.

Please keep eyes closed when taking this steam; these particular essential oils may sting the eyes or cause excessive tearing.

Delicate Flower Express Steam

This steam is designed especially for delicate, thin, damaged skin lacking in vitality, suppleness, and tone.

3 cups distilled water
4 drops neroli essential oil
2 drops frankincense essential oil (CO_2 extract)

RECOMMENDED FOR: *normal, dry, sensitive, mature, or environmentally damaged skin (except for those types listed in Contraindications on page 165)*
USE: *1 or 2 times per week*
FOLLOW WITH: *moisturizer*
PREP TIME: *approximately 5 minutes*
STORE IN: *do not store; mix as needed*
YIELD: *1 treatment*

PREPARATION AND APPLICATION TIPS: Follow general directions on page 165.

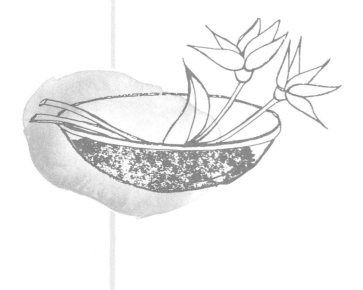

Exfoliant Facial Scrubs

A cosmetic facial scrub or *exfoliant* is used to remove dry, dead skin cells from the surface of the skin. Unlike many commercial facial scrubs that contain harsh, gritty pumice, ground apricot kernels, or walnut hulls; the recipes here contain softer, soothing ingredients that accomplish the same goal while being much easier on the skin.

Many women, especially those who wear minimal or no makeup, prefer to use a facial scrub instead of a foaming or cream or lotion cleanser for daily cleaning. The scrubs here cleanse, exfoliate, and nourish and never strip protective oils from the skin.

Why exfoliate on a regular basis? Gentle, consistent exfoliation is essential to aid in cell turnover, revealing a fresher, smoother complexion that will more readily accept healing hydration from a toner, astringent, facial steam, mask, or moisturizer.

CONTRAINDICATIONS: Generally, scrubs can be used on all skin types *except* those with acne or acne rosacea; broken capillaries or thread veins; sensitive and irritated skin; thin, mature, or elderly skin; or sunburned or windburned skin. If you do suffer from one or more of these "challenged" skin conditions, take heart; a couple of recipes offered here are very gentle yet effective and can help improve the look and feel of your skin.

APPLICATION TIPS: When using any of these exfoliants, especially the more granular ones, *do not scrub your face and neck.* They are

SKIN REGENERATION

According to Dr. Peter T. Pugliese, author of *Physiology of the Skin* (Allured Publishing, 1996), the epidermis is able to replace itself completely in 45 to 74 days. In young people, the *stratum corneum* (the skin's outermost and hardest layer) can be fully replaced in about 14 days. This layer can take as long as 37 days to be replaced in people 50 and older.

not the kitchen sink! Your body may be able to tolerate a bit more friction from body brushes, loofahs, and sugar or salt scrubs, but your more delicate face and neck skin tissue will not tolerate such rough handling. Please allow the product to do the work for you and be very gentle, avoiding the eye area at all times! If you wear heavy makeup or foundation; if your skin is laden with work-related liquid vegetable, hydrogenated, or petroleum-based oils and grease; or if you've just finished a day of yard and gardening work; remove this layer of filth first with your usual cleanser, then proceed with the facial scrub.

ALL-PURPOSE SCRUB

This recipe was the very first skin care product I ever made. I was about 15 at the time and I've used and loved it ever since. It leaves skin feeling very smooth and doubles as a facial mask: Simply leave on and allow to dry for 20 minutes, then rinse.

½ cup ground oatmeal

¼ cup almond meal

¼ cup sunflower seed meal

1 teaspoon ground peppermint, spearmint, or rosemary leaves

Dash cinnamon powder (optional, but adds a hint of exotic fragrance)

Purified water (for oily skin), milk (for normal skin), or cream (for dry skin)

RECOMMENDED FOR: *all skin types (except those types listed in Contraindications on page 175)*
USE: *daily or as needed*
FOLLOW WITH: *moisturizer*
PREP TIME: *approximately 10 minutes (if meals are ground ahead of time)*
BLENDING TOOLS: *small bowl and spoon or whisk or plastic bag; bowl and spoon or whisk to mix scrub for use*
STORE IN: *zip-seal bag, plastic or glass jar, or tin (dry ingredients only)*
YIELD: *approximately 1 cup dry ingredients*

In a small bowl, thoroughly blend all dry ingredients using a spoon or small whisk, or shake them in a zip-seal plastic bag.

Pour the mixture into a storage container.

No refrigeration is required for dry ingredients, but for maximum freshness and potency, please use within 6 months.

TO MIX THE SCRUB FOR USE: In a small bowl, combine 2–3 teaspoons of dry scrub mixture for the face (or more of you plan to use it on your body) with enough water (for oily skin), milk (for normal skin), or cream (for dry skin) to form a spreadable paste. Allow the paste to thicken for 1 minute.

APPLICATION TIPS: Using your fingers, massage scrub onto face and throat. Rinse.

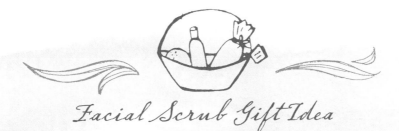

Facial Scrub Gift Idea

Facial scrub blends make great gifts for men or women.

- Make up a cup or two of the scrub (dry ingredients only) that best suits the recipient's skin type.
- Put it in a plastic freezer bag and tie the bag with a ribbon or twine.
- Place it in a decorative tin, box, or gift bag, along with complete instructions for making the scrub, a small condiment mixing bowl, and a set of pretty measuring spoons.
- Including a bottle of herbal hydrosol to blend with the scrub is a luxurious addition to the gift!

GENTLE FACIAL EXFOLIANT

*T*his scrub doubles as a facial mask: Simply apply and let dry for 20 minutes, then rinse.

½ cup ground oatmeal
¼ cup powdered milk, whole or nonfat
1 teaspoon cornmeal
Purified water

RECOMMENDED FOR: *all skin types, especially dry (except those types listed in Contraindications on page 175). If you omit the cornmeal, then any skin type can use it.*
USE: *daily or as needed*
FOLLOW WITH: *moisturizer*
PREP TIME: *approximately 5 minutes (if oatmeal is ground ahead of time)*
BLENDING TOOLS: *small bowl and spoon or whisk or plastic bag; bowl and spoon or whisk to mix scrub for use*
STORE IN: *zip-seal bag, plastic or glass jar, or tin (dry ingredients only)*
YIELD: *approximately ¾ cup dry ingredients*

In a small bowl, thoroughly blend all dry ingredients using a spoon or small whisk, or shake them in a sealed plastic bag.

Pour the mixture into a storage container.

No refrigeration is required for dry ingredients, but for maximum freshness and potency, please use within 6 months.

TO MIX THE SCRUB FOR USE: In a small bowl combine 1 tablespoon of scrub mixture with enough water to form a spreadable paste. Allow the mixture to thicken for 1 minute.

APPLICATION TIPS: Using your fingers, massage scrub onto the face and throat. Rinse.

SCRUB FOR OILY SKIN

*T*his scrub is great for oily areas on the shoulders, chest, and back. It doubles as a
mask: Simply apply and leave on to dry for 20 minutes, then rinse.

½ cup ground oatmeal

½ cup almond meal

1 tablespoon sea salt,
finely ground

1 teaspoon ground
peppermint leaves

1 teaspoon ground
rosemary leaves

Astringent of choice

RECOMMENDED FOR: *oily, combination, normal,
and oily mature skin (except those types listed in
Contraindications on page 175)*
USE: *2 times per week*
FOLLOW WITH: *moisturizer*
PREP TIME: *approximately 10 minutes (if meals are
ground ahead of time)*
BLENDING TOOLS: *small bowl and spoon or whisk
or plastic bag; bowl and spoon or whisk to mix scrub
for use*
STORE IN: *zip-seal bag, plastic or glass jar, or tin
(dry ingredients only)*
YIELD: *1 heaping cup dry ingredients*

In a small bowl, thoroughly blend all dry ingredients using a spoon
or small whisk, or shake them in a sealed plastic bag.

Pour the mixture into a storage container.

No refrigeration is required for dry ingredients, but for maximum freshness and potency, please use within 6 months.

TO MIX THE SCRUB FOR USE: In a small bowl, combine 1 tablespoon of scrub for the face (or more if you plan to use it on the body) with enough astringent to form a spreadable paste. Allow the mixture to thicken for 1 minute.

APPLICATION TIPS: Using your fingers, gently massage scrub onto the face and throat. Rinse.

CREAMY SCRUB CLEANSER

If this scrub is used frequently, your skin will acquire a "peaches and cream" glow. This very hydrating and moisturizing scrub doubles as a moisturizing mask: Simply apply and recline for 20 minutes, then rinse. It may be a bit runny, so to use it as a mask, don a shower cap or wrap your hair in a towel.

¼ small, ripe peach, peeled	RECOMMENDED FOR: *normal, dry, sensitive, environmentally damaged, and mature skin (except those types listed in Contraindications on page 175)*
1 tablespoon cream, light or heavy (or 2 tablespoons cream if peach is unavailable)	USE: *daily or as needed*
	FOLLOW WITH: *moisturizer*
1 tablespoon ground oatmeal	PREP TIME: *approximately 5 to 10 minutes (if meals are ground ahead of time)*
1 teaspoon chamomile flowers, powdered	BLENDING TOOLS: *mortar and pestle or small bowl and fork*
1 teaspoon sunflower seed meal	STORE IN: *do not store; mix as needed*
	YIELD: *1 treatment*

Using a mortar and pestle or a small bowl and fork, mash the peach until smooth. Mix all ingredients together with the peach to form a very creamy paste. If too thin, add more ground oats; if too thick, add more cream. Allow to thicken 1 minute.

APPLICATION TIPS: Using your fingers, massage scrub onto the face, throat, and décolleté (if desired). Allow the mixture to remain on your face for approximately 5 minutes. Rinse.

ALMOND MEAL CLEANSER

*T*his is a very basic and quickly made scrub. When a larger quantity of the almond meal is blended with milk or cream, it makes an excellent, delicious, nutty cereal, too!

2 teaspoons almond meal
Purified water (for oily skin),
    milk (for normal skin),
    or cream (for dry skin)

RECOMMENDED FOR: *all skin types (except those types listed in Contraindications on page 175)*
USE: *daily or as needed*
FOLLOW WITH: *moisturizer*
PREP TIME: *approximately 5 minutes (if meal is ground ahead of time)*
BLENDING TOOLS: *small bowl and spoon*
STORE IN: *do not store; mix as needed*
YIELD: *1 treatment*

In a small bowl, combine the almond meal with enough water (for oily skin), milk (for normal skin), or cream (for dry skin) to form a spreadable paste. Allow the mixture to thicken for 1 minute.

APPLICATION TIPS: Using your fingers, spread onto moistened face and throat and gently massage for 1 minute. Rinse.

Oatmeal Smoother

This scrub, gentle enough for a baby's delicate skin, leaves skin very smooth and soft. It doubles as a mask: Simply apply and leave on to dry for 20 to 30 minutes, then rinse._

½ cup ground oatmeal
½ cup powdered milk
Purified water

RECOMMENDED FOR: _all skin types, no exceptions (it is only minimally abrasive)_
USE: _daily or as desired_
FOLLOW WITH: _moisturizer_
PREP TIME: _approximately 5 minutes (if oatmeal is ground ahead of time)_
BLENDING TOOLS: _small bowl and spoon or whisk or plastic bag; bowl and spoon or whisk to mix scrub for use_
STORE IN: _zip-seal bag, plastic or glass jar, or tin (dry ingredients only)_
YIELD: _1 cup dry ingredients_

In a small bowl, thoroughly mix dry ingredients using a spoon or small whisk or shake them in a sealed plastic bag.

Pour the mixture into a storage container.

No refrigeration is required for the dry ingredients, but for maximum freshness and potency, please use within 6 months.

To mix scrub, combine 2 teaspoons of scrub mixture with 1 to 2 teaspoons water until a spreadable paste forms. Adjust water quantity as necessary. Allow the mixture to thicken for 1 minute.

APPLICATION TIPS: Using your fingers, massage onto face and throat. Rinse.

BALANCING SCRUB AND SKIN LIGHTENER

This scrub serves as a skin lightener to balance uneven or blotchy tone. The papain or enzyme in the papaya pulp acts as a chemical exfoliant, dissolving dead skin cells, leaving skin with an ultra-smooth appearance. If you choose to use plain yogurt instead of papaya, its lactic acid acts in a similar manner. For greater skin lightening results, use the recipe as an exfoliating mask: Eliminate the sugar and apply as you would the scrub, but leave on for 20 to 30 minutes as you recline and relax, then rinse. The mixture may be a bit runny, so to use it as a mask, don a shower cap or wrap your hair in a towel.

1 tablespoon papaya pulp or plain yogurt

2–3 teaspoons ground oatmeal (more for thicker consistency)

1 teaspoon sugar, finely granulated

RECOMMENDED FOR: *oily, combination, normal, and mature skin (except those types listed in Contraindications on page 175). If you omit the sugar, then all skin types except very sensitive or irritated skin can use this minimally abrasive scrub.*

USE: *2 times per week if well tolerated*

FOLLOW WITH: *moisturizer*

PREP TIME: *approximately 5 to 10 minutes (if oatmeal is ground ahead of time)*

BLENDING TOOLS: *mortar and pestle or small bowl and fork*

STORE IN: *do not store; mix as needed*

YIELD: *1 treatment*

Using a mortar and pestle or a small bowl and fork, combine ingredients until a spreadable paste forms. Allow the mixture to thicken for 1 minute.

APPLICATION TIPS: Using your fingers, lightly massage mixture onto the face, throat, and décolleté for 1 minute. Leave on for 5 minutes. Rinse with cool water.

SENSATIONAL SUNFLOWER FRICTION

The malic acid in the apple juice in this scrub helps to refine the skin's surface and chemically remove dead skin cells. The mixture is very hydrating and excellent to use regularly if you live or work in an arid environment. This scrub is a bit runny, so don a shower cap or wrap your hair in a towel before use.

1 tablespoon sunflower seed meal

1 tablespoon applesauce

RECOMMENDED FOR: *normal, dry, dehydrated, sensitive, environmentally damaged, and mature skin (except those types listed in Contraindications on page 175)*
USE: *2 or 3 times per week*
FOLLOW WITH: *moisturizer*
PREP TIME: *approximately 5 minutes (if meal is ground ahead of time)*
BLENDING TOOLS: *small bowl and spoon*
STORE IN: *do not store; mix as needed*
YIELD: *1 treatment*

In a small bowl, combine ingredients to form a spreadable paste. Allow the mixture to thicken for 1 minute.

APPLICATION TIPS: Using your fingers, massage onto the face, throat, and décolleté (if desired). Lie down and leave the mask on for 10 minutes so that the oils of the sunflower seed meal can be absorbed by your thirsty skin. Rinse.

PINEAPPLE-SUNFLOWER SCRUB

*D*ue to the natural acids in the pineapple or lemon juice, this scrub tends to bleach the skin slightly and act as a chemical exfoliant. Use it every week until your skin takes on a smooth, more balanced, even-toned appearance. This scrub is a bit runny, so don a shower cap or wrap your hair in a towel before use.*

1   tablespoon fresh, raw pineapple juice from fruit (or substitute lemon juice diluted 50 percent with water)

1   tablespoon sunflower seed meal

RECOMMENDED FOR: *oily, combination, normal, environmentally damaged, and oily mature skin (except those types listed in Contraindications on page 175)*
USE: *2 times per week if well tolerated*
FOLLOW WITH: *moisturizer*
PREP TIME: *approximately 5 to 10 minutes (if meal is ground ahead of time)*
BLENDING TOOLS: *mortar and pestle, small bowl and spoon*
STORE IN: *do not store; mix as needed*
YIELD: *1 treatment*

If using pineapple juice, mash a small amount of fresh, peeled fruit using a mortar and pestle, then strain the juice. In a small bowl, combine ingredients to form a spreadable paste. Adjust the amount of liquid to make the desired consistency.

APPLICATION TIPS: Using your fingers, massage onto the face, throat, and décolleté (if desired). Allow to remain on skin for 10 minutes. Rinse.

Cornmeal and Honey Scrub

This product leaves skin smooth, soft, and very hydrated. Because this scrub can be a bit runny and sticky, don a shower cap or wrap your hair in a towel before use.

1½ teaspoons cornmeal
1 teaspoon honey
½ teaspoon water

RECOMMENDED FOR: *all skin types (except those types listed in Contraindications on page 175)*
USE: *2 times per week*
FOLLOW WITH: *moisturizer if needed*
PREP TIME: *approximately 5 minutes*
BLENDING TOOLS: *small bowl and spoon*
STORE IN: *do not store; mix as needed*
YIELD: *1 treatment*

In a small bowl, combine ingredients thoroughly and allow cornmeal to absorb liquids for 1 minute.

APPLICATION TIPS: Using your fingers, gently massage onto the face and throat, lie back, and leave on for 15 minutes. Rinse with warm water.

BREWER'S YEAST AND OATMEAL SCRUB

This scrub really revs up the circulation — it restores life and glow to the complexion.

¼ cup brewer's yeast
¼ cup ground oatmeal
Purified water

RECOMMENDED FOR: *all skin types except dry or dehydrated skin*
USE: *2 times per week*
FOLLOW WITH: *moisturizer*
PREP TIME: *approximately 5 minutes (if oatmeal is ground ahead of time)*
BLENDING TOOLS: *small bowl and spoon or whisk or plastic bag; bowl and spoon or whisk to mix scrub for use*
STORE IN: *zip-seal bag, plastic or glass jar, or tin (dry ingredients only)*
YIELD: *½ cup dry ingredients*

In a small bowl, mix dry ingredients using a spoon or tiny whisk or shake them in a sealed plastic bag.

No refrigeration is required for dry ingredients, but for maximum freshness and potency, please use within 6 months.

TO THE MIX SCRUB FOR USE: In a small bowl, combine 1 table-spoon scrub with enough water to form a spreadable paste. Allow mixture to thicken for 1 minute.

APPLICATION TIPS: Using your fingers, massage onto the face and throat and allow to dry for 15 minutes. Rinse with cool water.

Tropical Enzyme Skin-Lightening Exfoliant

*I*f used repeatedly, this treatment will lighten skin discolorations or hyperpigmentation and will generally brighten a lackluster complexion. It's effective to use on sun-damaged, blotchy skin.

A few tablespoons fresh, raw papaya or pineapple (*Note:* Juice must be raw and fresh; "cooked" or pasteurized juices do not contain the necessary live, skin-brightening enzymes.)

RECOMMENDED FOR: *all skin types, especially those for whom granular scrubs are not indicated (but avoid if skin is very sensitive, irritated, sunburned, or windburned)*
USE: *1 or 2 times per week as tolerated*
FOLLOW WITH: *moisturizer*
PREP TIME: *approximately 5 to 10 minutes*
BLENDING TOOLS: *mortar and pestle, strainer*
STORE IN: *do not store; mix as needed*
YIELD: *1 treatment*

Using a mortar and pestle, mash a small piece of either type of fruit until smooth and pulpy. Strain the pulp until you have approximately 1 tablespoon of juice.

APPLICATION TIPS: Saturate a cotton ball or cotton square with fruit juice and apply to the face, throat, and décolleté in upward strokes until the area is completely covered by a thin layer of juice. Allow the juice to dry for 10 minutes. Rinse with cool water.

Note: It's normal to feel a slight tingle or stinging sensation as the juice dries; this simply means the fruit acids and protein-dissolving enzymes in the juice are doing their job digesting dead skin-dulling cell debris and brightening your complexion. If the feeling becomes uncomfortable, however, rinse immediately with cool water. Your skin may be too sensitive for this treatment.

Smooth-as-Silk Oatmeal Exfoliant, Cleanser, and Mask

*T*his is a perfect basic, multipurpose cosmetic. It can be left on the skin for 20 minutes to dry as a mask for all skin types; in a larger quantity it can be used as an effective, soap-free daily cleanser for the face or entire body; and it can be used as an extremely gentle scrub. It travels well, needs no preservatives, and won't spoil. What more could you ask?

1 tablespoon oat flour or very finely ground oatmeal

Hydrosol of choice or purified water

RECOMMENDED FOR: *all skin types, no exceptions*
USE: *daily if desired*
FOLLOW WITH: *moisturizer*
PREP TIME: *approximately 5 minutes (if oatmeal is ground ahead of time)*
BLENDING TOOLS: *small bowl and spoon*
STORE IN: *do not store; mix as needed*
YIELD: *1 treatment*

In a small bowl, combine the oat flour or fine oatmeal with enough of chosen liquid to form a smooth, spreadable paste. Allow the mixture to thicken for 1 minute. Add more liquid if it's too thick or more oats if it's too thin.

APPLICATION TIPS: Using your fingers, massage onto the face, throat, and décolleté. Rinse.

MICRODERMABRASION

Microdermabrasion is a professional skin care service that literally means abrasion or polishing of the skin using very tiny crystals. Most often this is done using a hand-held device that "sand blasts" the skin with a type of micronized crystal, frequently very fine aluminum. You'll find this expensive, popular service offered by many of today's better salons and spas. When performed correctly, this procedure, repeated over several weeks time, can aid in erasing or diminishing fine lines, wrinkles, and age spots and restore a smoothness and even texture to the skin that you may not have seen in quite some time.

Microdermabrasion is often recommended for those whose skin suffers from hyperpigmentation and environmental damage. However, if the technician is not trained properly or educated in appropriate skin care, uncomfortable damage can result with the removal of too much of the skin's outer surface, leaving it quite red and irritated. Even if this visible damage does not occur, wear sunscreen at all times following treatment and observe common sun sense, even on cloudy days, because the skin's protective shield has been compromised and thinned.

As a licensed esthetician, I'm often privy to industry trends and trade secrets used by high-end, luxury spas and promoted by them as "exclusive." Sometimes their "secret" ingredients are so inexpensive and their products are so simple to create that it's appalling how much such spas charge for their products and services. This manual microdermabrasion (sans machine) recipe is one of these "exclusive" secrets — and it costs only pennies per treatment. In addition, it's safer and won't ever leave your skin red or irritated, because of gentle hand application. If this treatment is used on a regular basis, your skin will achieve almost the same results as mechanical microdermabrasion, without having its protective shield compromised.

Manual Microdermabrasion

1   tablespoon baking soda
1½   teaspoons water
2   drops helichrysum essential oil

RECOMMENDED FOR: *all skin types except sunburned, windburned, or irritated skin*
USE: *1 or 2 times per week*
FOLLOW WITH: *moisturizer*
PREP TIME: *approximately 5 minutes*
BLENDING TOOLS: *small bowl and spoon*
STORE IN: *do not store; mix as needed*
YIELD: *1 treatment*

In a small bowl, combine all ingredients until a velvety slurry (watery paste) forms.

APPLICATION TIPS: Dip the pads of your fingers into the slurry and slowly and lightly begin to massage the entire face, throat, and décolleté, using very small, circular motions. Do not use much pressure — let the tiny baking soda granules do the exfoliation work. Continue to dip fingers into the baking soda mixture as often as needed in order to cover skin with a thin coat. The procedure takes almost 10 minutes to complete. Rinse.

Basic Clay Exfoliant, Cleanser, and Mask

This is another perfect, basic, multipurpose cosmetic. It can be left on the skin for 20 minutes to dry as a mask for oily, combination, and normal skin; in a larger quantity it can be used as an effective, soap-free cleanser for the face or entire body; and it can be used as an extremely gentle scrub. It travels well, needs no preservatives, and won't spoil.

1   tablespoon white clay
Hydrosol of choice or
     purified water

RECOMMENDED FOR: *all skin types, no exceptions*
USE: *daily if desired*
FOLLOW WITH: *moisturizer*
PREP TIME: *approximately 5 minutes*
BLENDING TOOLS: *small bowl and spoon*
STORE IN: *do not store; mix as needed*
YIELD: *1 treatment*

In a small bowl, combine the clay and about 1 teaspoon of chosen liquid to form a smooth, spreadable paste. Allow the mixture to thicken for 1 minute.

APPLICATION TIPS: Using your fingers, massage onto the face, throat, and décolleté. Rinse.

Face Moisturizers

Moisturizers can be your skin's best friend. By applying one, you are, in effect, putting a barrier between your skin and a world full of pollutants; dehydrating indoor heat and air-conditioning; and potential age-accelerating, damaging environmental factors. Moisturizers soothe, protect, coat, and promote suppleness.

Depending upon the skin type for which the moisturizer is created, varying quantities and types of water-based and oil-based ingredients are used. Always use a moisturizer designed for your skin type to avoid skin that appears oily from overmoisturizing or that is thirsty from undermoisturizing.

"COOKING" TIPS: Please read the general "cooking" tips detailed under Face Cleansers on page 111 before you proceed with the following recipes.

STORAGE TIPS: The moisturizing creams and lotions here contain no preservatives, thus they have a short shelf life. They require no refrigeration if used within 30 days unless the weather is very warm. If a homemade moisturizing cream is stored in the refrigerator unopened, then it may last up to 6 months. Refrigeration may unfavorably change the product's consistency, but its potency will be preserved. Herbal elixirs do not require refrigeration if used within 3 to 6 months unless your storage area is very warm.

APPLICATION TIPS: Unless otherwise specified, creams and herbal elixirs should always be applied to freshly cleansed skin following the use of your favorite toner, astringent, or hydrosol and immediately following any facial treatment such as a scrub, steam, or mask.

Don't forget to moisturize your neck and décolleté (chest, if you're a man). Many women (and most men) neglect these areas, which can actually reveal the aging effects of sun exposure and chronological years sooner than your face.

Light Moisturizer

Use this very light, hydrating moisturizer any time skin needs refreshing or is feeling tight and dry. The glycerin acts as a skin-softening humectant, drawing moisture from the air to the skin.

½ cup distilled water

2 teaspoons vegetable glycerin

5 drops lemon, geranium, grapefruit, or rosemary (chemotype *verbenon*) essential oil

RECOMMENDED FOR: *all skin types, especially oily, combination, normal, sunburned, windburned, or dehydrated skin*
USE: *daily*
PREP TIME: *approximately 5 minutes*
BLENDING TOOLS: *shake before each use*
STORE IN: *plastic or glass bottle or spritzer*
YIELD: *slightly more than ½ cup*

Add ingredients to a storage container and shake vigorously to blend.

No refrigeration is required, but for maximum freshness and potency, please use within 6 months.

APPLICATION TIPS: This product can be applied to face and throat with a cotton pad or by spraying the skin lightly and allowing to dry.

Aloe and Calendula Cleansing Cream

This is one of my favorite all-purpose herbal creams. It serves as an effective light- to medium-weight moisturizer for the face and body. I use it as a cleanser and moisturizer when the weather is cool and dry and I need a bit more oil in my skin.

See recipe under Face Cleansers, pages 114–115.

Whether used as a cleanser or a moisturizer, it's ideal for normal, dry, mature, sensitive, or environmentally damaged skin and is absorbed quickly without leaving an oily residue.

APPLICATION TIPS: Apply cream to face, throat, décolleté, body — anywhere that needs a little moisture!

Lemony Whip Cleansing Cream

I use this cream as a cleanser and moisturizer when the weather is warm and humid and my skin is pumping out a bit too much of its natural oil. Like the Aloe and Calendula Cleaning Cream above, this one also serves as an effective light- to medium-weight moisturizer for the face and body.

See recipe under Face Cleansers, pages 124–125.

Whether used as a cleanser or a moisturizer, it's ideal for oily, combination, and normal skin, and is absorbed quickly without leaving an oily residue.

APPLICATION TIPS: Apply cream to face, throat, décolleté, and body as needed throughout the day to control shine.

Cocoa Butter Creamy Lotion for Face and Body

*T*his nongreasy, deeply moisturizing and hydrating cream doubles as a fabulous after-sun cream. It leaves skin very soft and silky with a light, velvety "orangesicle" scent.

7	tablespoons soybean, almond, apricot kernel, or macadamia nut base oil
2	tablespoons beeswax
2	tablespoons coconut base oil (extra-virgin, unrefined)
1	tablespoon cocoa butter
1	teaspoon anhydrous lanolin
9	tablespoons distilled water
2	teaspoons vegetable glycerin
½	teaspoon borax
30	drops sweet orange essential oil
20	drops tangerine or sweet orange essential oil
20	drops vanilla essential oil

RECOMMENDED FOR: *normal, dry, dehydrated, sensitive, sunburned, windburned, mature, or environmentally damaged skin (especially for dehydrated oily and combination skin in cooler, less humid seasons)*
USE: *daily*
PREP TIME: *approximately 20 to 30 minutes, plus 30 minutes to set up and cool*
BLENDING TOOLS: *blender; long-handled, slender spatula*
STORE IN: *glass or plastic jars or squeeze bottle (if storage area is very warm)*
YIELD: *approximately 1⅓ cups*

HEAT: In a small saucepan over low heat or in a double boiler, warm the base oils, beeswax, cocoa butter, and lanolin, until the cocoa butter and beeswax are just melted. In another pan, warm the water and vegetable glycerin, add the borax, and stir until the borax is incorporated.

COOL: Remove both pans from heat and allow their contents to cool almost to body temperature, until the oils/wax/butter/lanolin mixture just begins to thicken and becomes slightly opaque. It will be like a soft, loose salve. This will take 5 to 10 minutes, depending on the temperature of your kitchen.

BLEND: Immediately pour the oils/wax/butter/lanolin mixture into the blender, scraping the sides of the saucepan to remove every last trace. Place the lid on the blender and remove the lid's plastic piece. Turn the blender on medium and slowly drizzle the water/glycerin/borax mixture through the center of the lid into the vortex of swirling fats below. Closely watch what happens: almost immediately, the lotion will begin to thicken. Blend for 5 to 10 seconds more, turn off the blender, and check the consistency. It should have a smooth texture. If the mixtures are not combining properly, turn off the blender and give the lotion a few manual stirs with a spatula to free up the blender blades. Then replace the lid and blend on medium for another 5 to 10 seconds. Repeat process as needed.

Turn off the blender and add the essential oils, stirring a few times to mix them in, then blend completely on medium another 5 to 10 seconds, until the lotion is smooth and pale yellow. *Note:* If the temperature of your kitchen is above 76°F, the lotion will maintain a softer consistency. (Coconut oil turns from solid to liquid at 76°F.) If the temperature is below 76°F, the lotion will be firmer, more like a cream.

PACKAGE AND COOL: Pour the finished lotion into storage container(s). Lightly cover each container with a paper towel and allow the lotion to cool for 30 minutes before capping. If you notice, after a few hours or days, that water begins to separate from the lotion, don't worry. The mixture can separate if the fat temperature and water temperature are not relatively equal and cool enough when the two portions are blended. Keep trying — crafting perfect lotions is an art form!

No refrigeration of this product is required if it's used within 30 days. If stored in the refrigerator, please use it within 3 to 6 months. (You may notice a change in the formula's texture if it's stored in the refrigerator, but this won't affect the quality of the product.)

APPLICATION TIPS: Use ½ to 1 teaspoon to cover the entire face, throat, and décolleté and more as necessary for the body.

Rich and Royal
Regeneration Flower Cream

This is an intensely fragrant, luxurious cream fit for a queen! Though the recipe makes only a small amount, a little goes a long way. The exotically aromatic essential oils and rose hip seed base oil are healing and nourishing and act as cellular regenerators. The natural and therapeutic floral essence of this cream transcends an irritating synthetic fragrance any day.

2   tablespoons almond, soybean, or macadamia nut base oil

2   teaspoons rose hip seed base oil

1½   teaspoons beeswax

1   tablespoon distilled water or rose, rose geranium, or neroli hydrosol

1   small vitamin E oil capsule (optional)

10   drops lavender or geranium essential oil

10   drops neroli essential oil

5–10 drops ylang ylang essential oil

RECOMMENDED FOR: *all skin types except oily or combination skin*
USE: *daily*
PREP TIME: *approximately 30 minutes, plus 1 hour to set and synergize*
BLENDING TOOLS: *small whisk or spoon*
STORE IN: *glass or plastic jar*
YIELD: *approximately ¼ cup*

HEAT: In a small saucepan over low heat or in a double boiler, warm the base oils and beeswax until the wax is just melted. In another pan, warm the water or hydrosol.

COOL: Remove both pans from heat and allow their contents to cool almost to body temperature, until the oils/wax mixture just begins to thicken but is still liquid.

BLEND: Quickly drizzle the hydrosol into the oils/wax mixture while stirring or whisking rapidly. (Unlike many of the other cream and lotion recipes here, this recipe doesn't require a blender, though an extra pair of hands is helpful at this juncture!) Continue rapidly stirring the cream for 2 to 4 minutes or until a pale-yellow emulsion forms. Pierce the vitamin E capsule (if using) and squeeze the contents into the cream, add the essential oils, and rapidly stir for another 4 or 5 minutes or until the mixture is cool. This recipe really gives your forearm a workout! You should now have a moderately thick, shiny cream.

PACKAGE AND COOL: Spoon cream into a beautiful storage container — it looks best in a cobalt-blue glass jar. The product should be cool enough to allow you to cap the jar immediately so none of the volatile, rejuvenating essential oil properties can escape into the air. Allow the cream to set and synergize, for about an hour prior to use. No refrigeration is required if the cream is used within 30 days. It will last for 3 to 6 months if refrigerated.

APPLICATION TIPS: This cream is highly concentrated; you'll need only a pea-sized amount to cover the face and throat and a little more to cover the décolleté and breasts if you wish. Before applying, first rub the cream between your palms to warm it, then massage it into the skin.

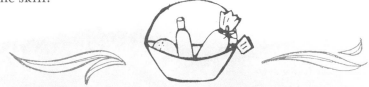

Face Moisturizer Gift Idea

Moisturizing creams and herbal elixirs are a welcome treat any time of the year, but especially during the summer and winter.

- Make up a fresh batch of moisturizer for a special friend.
- Put it in an attractive glass or plastic container.
- Attach a label or tag with complete instructions for use and the expiration date.
- Wrap it in tissue paper and place it in a small gift bag.
- You can also include a pair of inexpensive cotton gloves or socks, especially if you make one of the heavier moisturizers that double as an overnight hand and foot conditioner.

Herbal Facial Elixirs

In the mid-1990s, I decided to see what all the hoopla was about concerning the highly touted "youthifying" commercial facial serums that many cosmetic companies were launching. These ½- to 1-ounce bottles of promise came at a hefty price, and after a bit of ingredient sleuthing on my part, I discovered that they consisted primarily of water, synthetic skin softeners, chemical exfoliating acids, a vitamin or two, humectants, artificial fragrance, and preservatives.

So I decided to create my own natural, highly beneficial versions of these serums. The result: herbal facial elixirs that your skin will literally drink! If used consistently, the elixirs here will definitely aid in prolonging the youthful qualities of your skin.

The prep time is quick, but plan on setting aside your elixir for one day. Have you ever heard the expression, "the sum is greater than its parts"? There's a scientific term for that, and it's *synergy*. During the 24 hours that you let your blend rest, you are letting it synergize, to become a more powerful conditioner for your skin.

Think of the following recipes as alternative moisturizing treatments for your face. Instead of applying a traditionally made cream or lotion, first moisten your skin with your favorite toner or astringent, then apply one of these specialized blends of pure base and essential oils. They'll nourish on a cellular level, restore, soften, balance, hydrate, and repair damaged skin. Expect visible results after regular use. As an added benefit, the aromatherapeutic properties of these elixirs will serve to calm, uplift, recharge, or soothe the mind and spirit.

Healing Thyme Elixir

This elixir helps to balance problem skin due to overactive sebaceous glands. The combination of essential oils produces an antiseptic, antibacterial formula that also calms the skin, counteracting redness from inflammation. It also aids in normalizing dry areas, improves sluggish circulation, and stimulates new cell formation.

5   drops rosemary
    (chemotype *verbenon*)
    essential oil

5   drops thyme (chemotype
    linalol) essential oil

2   drops lemon essential oil

8   drops German
    chamomile essential oil

2   tablespoons
    hazelnut base oil

RECOMMENDED FOR: *oily, acneic (with weeping acne), combination, or normal skin*
USE: *2 times per day*
PREP TIME: *approximately 15 minutes, plus 24 hours to synergize*
BLENDING TOOLS: *shake storage bottle prior to each use*
STORE IN: *dark glass bottle with glass dropper top*
YIELD: *2 tablespoons or 1 ounce*

Add the essential oils, drop by drop, directly into a storage bottle. Next, add the base oil. Screw on the dropper bottle top, wrap your hand around the bottle, and shake the formula vigorously for 2 minutes to completely blend all ingredients and gently warm them to body temperature.

Set the bottle in a dark location that's between 60 and 80°F for 24 hours so that the oils can synergize.

No refrigeration is required, but for maximum freshness and potency, please use within 6 months.

APPLICATION TIPS: Morning and evening after cleansing, apply the appropriate toner, astringent, or hydrosol. While skin is still damp, lightly massage 3 to 5 drops of elixir into skin, beginning with décolleté, throat, then face, using upward, outward, and circular strokes. Wait 5 minutes before applying sunscreen, additional moisturizer, or makeup.

Repair and Restore Elixir

This is a regenerative and anti-inflammatory elixir containing skin-supportive fatty acids that helps repair and pamper environmentally stressed and mature skin, leaving behind a healthy feel, more even tone, and suppleness. This blend can also be used to help prevent stretch marks, to speed post-operative skin healing and regeneration, and to aid in healing mild, first-degree burns.

7 drops carrot seed essential oil

7 drops helichrysum essential oil

6 drops calendula essential oil (CO_2 extract)

1 teaspoon rose hip seed base oil

1 teaspoon calophyllum base oil

1 teaspoon macadamia nut base oil

1 tablespoon apricot kernel base oil

RECOMMENDED FOR: *normal, dry, mature, sensitive, sunburned, windburned, or environmentally damaged skin; also for scarred skin tissue*
USE: *2 times per day (3 times per day for treatment of minor kitchen burns or sunburn)*
PREP TIME: *approximately 15 minutes, plus 24 hours to synergize*
BLENDING TOOLS: *shake storage bottle before each use*
STORE IN: *dark glass bottle with glass dropper top*
YIELD: *2 tablespoons or 1 ounce*

Add the essential oils, drop by drop, directly into storage bottle, then add the base oils. Screw on the dropper bottle top, wrap your hand around the bottle, and shake the formula vigorously for 2 minutes to completely blend all ingredients and gently warm them to body temperature.

Set the bottle in a dark location that's between 60 and 80°F for 24 hours so that the oils can synergize.

No refrigeration is required, but for maximum freshness and potency, please use within 6 months.

APPLICATION TIPS: Morning and evening after cleansing, apply the appropriate toner, astringent, or hydrosol. While skin is still very damp, place 3 to 5 drops of elixir into your palm, rub both palms together, and lightly massage the elixir into skin, beginning with the décolleté, throat, then face, using upward, outward, and circular strokes. Wait five minutes before applying sunscreen, additional moisturizer if desired, or makeup.

TO HELP PREVENT STRETCH MARKS AND THE RESULTING SCARS: Apply a combination of 1 teaspoon of rose hip seed base oil and 1 drop of calendula essential oil (CO_2 extract) directly to the expanding abdomen. Massage the entire area twice daily. *These are very safe oils,* but check with your physician first if you are concerned.

TO HELP PREVENT SCAR TISSUE AND SPEED HEALING: *Please consult with your physician prior to usage.* To help fade scar tissue that already exists, this elixir can be applied by the drop twice daily directly to scars anywhere on the body. Scars that are less than two years old will tend to respond more favorably than older scar tissue.

TO AID THE HEALING PROCESS OF BURNS: Use on burns that are not too severe and don't require a physician's care, including sunburns, grease burns, and general "kitchen accident" burns. Immediately pour chilled aloe vera juice onto the area to stop inflammation and cool the tissue. Follow this with an application of several drops of this elixir. Repeat this procedure up to 3 times per day. You should see dramatic improvement and recovery.

"There is a case for keeping wrinkles. They are the long-service stripes earned in the hard campaign of life."

— EDITORIAL IN THE *London Daily Mail*

Oh-So-Sensitive Elixir

This elixir is designed for very sensitive, weather-beaten, red, dry, and irritated skin. The base oils are nourishing, conditioning, protective, and highly absorptive. Every one of the essential oils is known for its calming, soothing, anti-inflammatory properties.

5 drops **each** of the following essential oils: German chamomile; calendula (CO2 extract); helichrysum; lavender

1 tablespoon jojoba base oil

1 teaspoon macadamia nut base oil

2 teaspoons sunflower base oil

RECOMMENDED FOR: *normal, dry, sensitive, mature, sunburned, windburned, or environmentally damaged skin, especially skin with broken surface capillaries and ruddiness*
USE: *2 times per day*
PREP TIME: *approximately 15 minutes, plus 24 hours to synergize*
BLENDING TOOLS: *shake storage bottle before each use*
STORE IN: *dark glass bottle with glass dropper top*
YIELD: *2 tablespoons or 1 ounce*

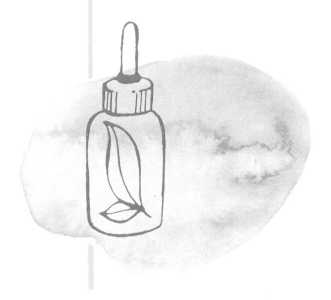

Add the essential oils, drop by drop, directly into a storage bottle. Next, add the base oils. Screw on the dropper bottle top, wrap your hand around the bottle, and shake the formula vigorously for 2 minutes to completely blend all ingredients and gently warm them to body temperature.

Set the bottle in a dark location that's between 60 and 80°F for 24 hours so that the oils can synergize.

No refrigeration is required, but for maximum freshness and potency, please use within 6 months.

APPLICATION TIPS: Morning and evening after cleansing, apply the appropriate toner, astringent, or hydrosol. While skin is still damp, lightly massage 3 to 5 drops of elixir into skin, beginning with the décolleté, throat, then face, using upward, outward, and circular strokes. Wait five minutes before applying sunscreen, additional moisturizer if desired, or makeup.

This elixir doubles as a calming treatment for irritations due to bug bites, poison plant exposure, diaper rash, eczema, psoriasis, and any contact dermatitis. For such use, apply by the drop twice daily.

"The flowers are nature's jewels, with whose wealth she decks her summer beauty."

— GEORGE CROLY, IRISH POET, AUTHOR, AND DIVINE

Evening Luxe Elixir

This elixir is designed for all skin types in need of light pampering and balancing. Hazelnut and jojoba base oils are compatible with human skin and will leave no oily residue. It softens, moisturizes, heals, rejuvenates, and tones the skin and speeds cell regeneration. Each of the essential oils has a calming, sedative effect on the psyche and body. Applying this just before bedtime can help lull you into restorative sleep.

8	drops neroli essential oil
4	drops frankincense essential oil (CO2 extract)
4	drops rose otto essential oil
4	drops lavender essential oil
1	tablespoon hazelnut base oil
1	tablespoon jojoba base oil

RECOMMENDED FOR: *all skin types*
USE: *1 time per day, right before bedtime*
PREP TIME: *approximately 15 minutes, plus 24 hours to synergize*
BLENDING TOOLS: *shake storage bottle before each use*
STORE IN: *dark glass bottle with glass dropper top*
YIELD: *2 tablespoons or 1 ounce*

Add the essential oils, drop by drop, directly into a storage bottle. Next, add the base oils. Screw on the dropper bottle top, wrap your hand around the bottle, and shake the formula vigorously for 2 minutes to completely blend all ingredients and gently warm them to body temperature.

Set bottle in a dark location that's between 60 and 80°F for 24 hours so that the oils can synergize.

No refrigeration is required, but for maximum freshness and potency, please use within 6 months.

APPLICATION TIPS: Immediately before bedtime and after cleansing your face, apply the appropriate toner, astringent, or hydrosol. While skin is still damp, lightly massage 3 to 5 drops of elixir into skin, beginning with the décolleté, throat, then face, using upward, outward, and circular strokes. Wait five minutes before applying additional moisturizer, if desired.

"Out Damn Spot" Antiblemish Elixir

This is a broad-spectrum antibacterial elixir specifically designed to zap subsurface acneic bacteria, ridding skin of toxins and associated redness. It's also excellent to use on infected ingrown hairs that can form after a bikini waxing or bikini-line shave.

4 drops tea tree essential oil	RECOMMENDED FOR: *any skin type with active blemishes*
2 drops clove essential oil	USE: *up to 2 times per day*
2 drops German chamomile essential oil	PREP TIME: *approximately 15 minutes, plus 24 hours to synergize*
2 drops green myrtle essential oil	BLENDING TOOLS: *shake storage bottle before each use*
2 teaspoons hazelnut or apricot kernel base oil	STORE IN: *dark glass bottle with glass dropper top*
1 teaspoon almond base oil	YIELD: *1 tablespoon or ½ ounce*

Add the essential oils, drop by drop, directly into storage bottle. Next, add the base oils. Screw on the dropper bottle top, wrap your hand around the bottle, and shake the formula vigorously for 2 minutes to completely blend all ingredients and gently warm them to body temperature.

Set the bottle in a dark location that's between 60 and 80°F for 24 hours so that the oils can synergize.

No refrigeration is required, but for maximum freshness and potency, please use within 6 months.

APPLICATION TIPS: Before applying, cleanse blemished area with either your regular cleanser or astringent or toner of choice. Then place 1 or 2 drops of elixir into your palm, dip a cotton swab into the oil, and dab onto each pesky pimple. Repeat up to 2 times per day.

TO USE ON INFECTED INGROWN HAIRS: Apply 1 drop to each hair removal area and massage in with your fingertips. Use 1 or 2 times per day. This product is also great for healing itchy bug bites.

Treatments for the Eyes

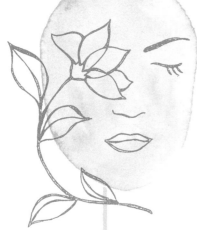

It's said that the eyes are the windows to the soul. But if you stay up nights with a crying, hungry infant, look at a computer screen all day, party hearty all night, sleep with your eyes squished into a pillow, spend time around smokers or in dry office air, have allergies, get makeup remover in your eyes, forget to remove your mascara at night, worship the sun, consume excess caffeine and not enough water, or regularly eat salty foods, your "windows" and their surrounding skin will look puffy, bloodshot, and irritated. They may even sting and tear. The tender eye area is one of the first places to give in to the formation of fine lines, wrinkles, and subsequent sagging. Yet natural remedies can come to the rescue to help soothe, brighten, depuff, and refresh those red and weary peepers. And remember — sleep is the best eye and beauty treatment of all!

Nighttime Eye Moisturizer

T *his simple treatment is highly moisturizing and softening and helps keep dry, crinkly wrinkles and laugh lines at bay. It's especially refreshing if the oil is chilled.*

¼ teaspoon jojoba, sesame, almond, extra-virgin olive, soybean, macadamia, avocado, or apricot kernel base oil

RECOMMENDED FOR: *combination, normal, dry, dehydrated, sensitive, environmentally damaged, or mature skin*
USE: *daily*
FOLLOW WITH: *moisturizer*
STORE IN: *follow package directions for base oil storage.*
YIELD: *1 treatment*

APPLICATION TIPS: Cleanse and tone your face and leave it slightly damp. Pour a few drops of chosen base oil into the palm of your hand — approximately ¼ teaspoon will do perfectly. Dip your ring finger into the oil and gently pat the substance around (not directly on) your eye in this fashion: Begin at the outer corner and slowly move beneath your eye toward the inner corner, then onto the very upper portion of the lid or brow bone area just below the actual brow, and back over to the outer corner. Do this several times, then pat off any excess oil, trying to leave a light film of oil on your skin. Follow this treatment with an application of your regular moisturizer to your face, neck, and décolleté.

Note: The reason for not applying the oil directly onto the lid and lashes is that if any of the oil were to get into your eye, it could potentially clog your tear ducts and cause puffiness (which we're trying to avoid!). The delicate eye area acts like a wick and will draw the moisture it needs from the surrounding moisturized tissue.

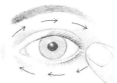

Eye Soothers

To help relieve puffiness and dark circles, apply any of the following to your eyes while reclining and resting for 15 minutes:

- Cold, damp black or green tea bags or cotton squares soaked in brewed, chilled tea of catnip, rose petals, chamomile flowers, elder flowers, eyebright, fennel seeds, lavender buds, or blackberry leaves
- Thin slices of cold cucumber or white potato
- Cold, witch hazel–soaked cotton pads
- Cold, whole milk–soaked cotton pads
- Chilled rose or lavender hydrosol — gentle enough to spritz directly into and around eyes or use as an eye wash
- Chilled, metal teaspoons; the cold temperature constricts blood vessels, decreasing puffiness, redness, and irritation. Place 4 teaspoons in ice water to chill. Leave two spoons chilling and take two spoons and apply one to each eye, concave side toward skin, following the contour of the eye socket. When spoons begin to warm, switch them with the spoons still chilling in the ice water. Continue, alternating spoons until puffiness subsides or for up to 20 minutes.

EYE RINSE

This treatment is very refreshing and soothing to tired, irritated, swollen eye tissue. It feels especially wonderful when the liquid is very cold — it actually perks you up physically and mentally.

1 cup distilled water
1 tablespoon eyebright, chamomile flowers, or crushed fennel seeds

RECOMMENDED FOR: *tired, dry, irritated, or bloodshot eyes*
USE: *as desired (if you wear contacts, remove them first before using product)*
PREP TIME: *approximately 45 minutes*
BLENDING TOOLS: *strainer; shake before each use*
STORE IN: *sterilized plastic or glass bottle or spritzer*
YIELD: *approximately 1 cup*

Bring the water to a boil and remove from heat. If using fennel seeds, crush them using a mortar and pestle. Add the herb of choice to the boiled water, cover, and steep for about 30 minutes. Strain the liquid twice through a nylon stocking or very fine cloth, or once through a coffee filter.

Pour into a sterilized storage container.

Refrigerate for up to 7 days, then discard.

APPLICATION TIPS: Either splash open eyes with the brew or lightly mist open eyes. An eye cup is also handy to use.

Eye Mask

This hydrates and tightens skin, diminishes puffiness, and leaves eyes feeling refreshed.

2	teaspoons cucumber or raw potato, peeled, seeded, and finely grated
1	teaspoon powdered milk

RECOMMENDED FOR: *puffy, baggy, tired eyes surrounded by dehydrated skin*
USE: *1 or 2 times per week*
FOLLOW WITH: *moisturizer*
PREP TIME: *approximately 35 minutes*
BLENDING TOOLS: *grater, mortar and pestle*
STORE IN: *do not store; mix as needed*
YIELD: *1 treatment*

Using a mortar and pestle, combine ingredients into a smooth, thick paste and chill for 30 minutes. Add a few drops of water if mixture needs to be thinned a bit.

APPLICATION TIPS: Lie down, close eyes, and apply mixture to the entire eye area, including the lids. Leave on for 10 minutes. Rinse with cool water.

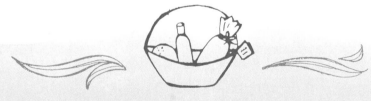

Eye Care Gift Idea

The Eye Rinse recipe makes a welcome gift for anyone who experiences frequent eye strain or lack of sleep. Pour a few ounces in a small, sterilized spritzer bottle, label, and tie a decorative ribbon around the top with instructions printed on an attractive gift card or parchment paper. Make sure to tell the lucky recipient to refrigerate it and use it within 7 days.

Lip Service: Luscious Lips

Unlike the rest of your skin, your lips do not contain any sebaceous glands (oil glands) or sweat glands to keep them moisturized and lubricated. Thus many of us constantly slather them with lipsticks, glosses, balms, and ointments of various kinds in an attempt to prevent drying and cracking and simultaneously keep them kissably soft and supple.

If you're a woman, you probably know from first hand experience that many brands of lipstick tend to be drying instead of moisturizing (regardless of the advertising hype). Some can even cause your lips to flake, peel, and become unsightly. What's more, I have yet to see an "all-day formula" that lasts past midmorning without becoming unattractively cakey. Yet take heart! Here you'll find two natural, moisturizing, lip-pampering formulas that you can make with or without color and one extra-rich formula that smells and tastes like vanilla-honey fudge. All ingredients used are actually edible — which is a good thing considering women tend to ingest several pounds of lipstick over a lifetime.

APPLICATION TIPS: The colorless versions can be worn alone or as a base or top coat with your favorite commercial lipstick. The colored versions contain no added drying chemicals or mica or fish scales for shimmer; nor do they have that metallic lipstick taste that can linger in your mouth for hours. These beeswax and honey formulas provide only a sheer wash of color.

Using these recipes, you can create a basic, nourishing lip balm or gloss that smells and tastes good, not synthetic or manufactured. Your children will enjoy these lip treats, too!

Healing and Cooling Lip Balm and Gloss

This lip treatment is rich, soothing, ultracooling, and especially good for lips that are weather–beaten or chapped and tender.

4–5 tablespoons almond, jojoba, soybean, or castor base oil (castor oil is preferred if you want a super-shiny gloss)

1 tablespoon beeswax

2 teaspoons honey

20 drops peppermint or spearmint essential oil or tea tree essential oil (optional)

½ tube of your favorite natural, synthetic-free, colored lipstick (optional)

RECOMMENDED FOR: *everyone*
USE: *as desired*
PREP TIME: *approximately 30 minutes plus 2 hours for flavor and consistency to synergize and set*
BLENDING TOOLS: *small whisk or spoon*
STORE IN: *small plastic or glass jars or tins*
YIELD: *approximately twelve to fourteen ¼-ounce containers or 6–7 tablespoons*

In a small saucepan over low heat or double boiler, warm oil, beeswax, and honey until the wax is just melted. Use 5 tablespoons of oil for a softer consistency; use 4 tablespoons for a firmer balm.

Remove from heat. Add the essential oil (if desired) and colored lipstick (if desired), and stir until the lipstick is melted. Set the pan in a shallow ice-water bath. Using a whisk or spoon, stir rapidly for 30 to 60 seconds until the honey is completely incorporated and the formula is like thick frosting. It will be a pale yellow color unless you've added colored lipstick.

Spoon the mixture into storage containers and cap. Let the mixture set for 2 hours before use.

No refrigeration is required, but for maximum freshness and taste, please use within 1 year.

Honey Fruit-Flavored Lip Balm

This balm is rich and soothing for year-round use. For great taste that appeals to children, you can flavor this balm with synthetic oils such as apple, apricot, peach, or cherry. Essential oils such as anise, fennel, or vanilla also add flavor. For the shiniest gloss, use castor oil as the base oil.

7–8 teaspoons almond, jojoba, soybean, or castor base oil

2 teaspoons beeswax

1 teaspoon honey

10 drops lemon, orange, lime, or tangerine essential oil (or oil or flavoring of choice)

¼ tube or less of your favorite natural, synthetic-free, colored lipstick (optional)

RECOMMENDED FOR: *everyone, especially children*
USE: *as desired*
PREP TIME: *approximately 30 minutes plus 2 hours for flavor and consistency to synergize and set*
BLENDING TOOLS: *small whisk or spoon*
STORE IN: *small plastic or glass jars or tins*
YIELD: *approximately 6–7 ¼-ounce containers or 3 heaping tablespoons*

In a small saucepan over low heat or double boiler, warm oil, beeswax, and honey until the wax is just melted. Use 8 teaspoons of oil for a softer consistency; use 7 teaspoons for a firmer balm.

Remove from heat. Add the essential oil or flavoring and the colored lipstick (if desired), and stir until the lipstick is melted. Set the pan in a shallow ice-water bath. Using a whisk or spoon, stir rapidly for 30 to 60 seconds until the honey is completely incorporated and the formula is like thick frosting. It will be a pale yellow color unless you've added colored lipstick.

Spoon the mixture into storage containers, and cap. Let the mixture set for 2 hours before use.

No refrigeration is required, but for maximum freshness and taste, please use within 1 year.

Simply Shiny Lip Gloss

Don't have time to create one of these silky, sweet lip treatment recipes? Simply apply a drop or two of pure castor oil to your lips for a thick, rich, high-gloss shine. Works in a pinch!

Rough Lip Scuff

This simple, lip-scuffing method quickly loosens flaky, dead skin, leaving lips smoother, softer, and healthier-looking. The brushing action stimulates circulation and actually causes lips to plump temporarily, improving the look of your sultry pout!

½ teaspoon baking soda
Premoistened toothbrush

RECOMMENDED FOR: *everyone, especially those who have chapped, rough, and weather-beaten lips*
USE: *as needed*
PREP TIME: *mere seconds*
BLENDING TOOLS: *toothbrush*
STORE IN: *do not store; mix as needed*
YIELD: *1 treatment*

Place baking soda into the palm of one hand and dip damp toothbrush bristles into the soda.

APPLICATION TIPS: Gently brush premoistened lips back and forth for approximately 20 seconds. Be careful not to brush too hard to avoid causing further irritation. Rinse.

Vanilla Velvet Honey Lip Balm

This rich and soothing balm can be used year-round. It doubles as a mild antibacterial ointment when applied to cuts and scrapes and helps prevent scarring.

1 tablespoon honey
1 tablespoon soybean or almond base oil
1 ½ teaspoons beeswax
5 drops vanilla essential oil

RECOMMENDED FOR: *everyone, especially children (flavor and texture are like vanilla honey fudge)*
USE: *as desired*
PREP TIME: *approximately 30 minutes, plus 2 hours for flavor and consistency to synergize and set*
BLENDING TOOLS: *small whisk or spoon*
STORE IN: *small plastic or glass jars or tins*
YIELD: *approximately five ¼-ounce containers or 2½ tablespoons*

In a small saucepan over low heat or in a double boiler, warm oil, honey, and beeswax, until the wax is just melted.

Remove from heat, add the essential oil, and stir to blend. Set the pan in a shallow ice-water bath. Using a whisk or spoon, stir rapidly for 30 to 60 seconds until the honey is incorporated and the formula is like thick peanut butter. It will be a pale yellow-brown color.

Spoon the mixture into storage containers and cap. Let the mixture set for 2 hours before use.

No refrigeration is required, but for maximum freshness and taste, please use within 1 year.

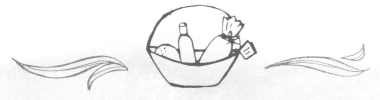

Lip Care Gift Idea

Many companies that retail herbs, essential oils, and other ingredients for the personal care crafter also sell various types of storage containers (see Resources on page 358 for a listing). I prefer to use the ¼-ounce plastic or glass jars or ½-ounce tins for soft balms and glosses instead of plastic tubes. A tube is ideal only for extra-firm, waxy balms. There are many styles of jars or tins to choose from — and these tiny sizes are perfect to hold all the flavors and colors of lip treats you wish to make as gifts or for yourself.

For gift-giving, lip treatments make great stocking stuffers at Christmas and can be an added bonus in a college-bound student's "care package" or a real necessity for someone going skiing in winter or vacationing in the tropics. Also, school-age children can carry a container in their purse, backpack, or jacket pocket.

Your Body Beautiful

The skin on your body, like the skin on your face, needs constant TLC in order to maintain its health, moisture content, smooth texture, resiliency, and comfort level as you age. Here you'll learn how to take care of your body beautiful naturally from the outside in. The recipes run the gamut from rich moisturizers and massage oils and bath treats such as fragrant oils, herbal bath bags, milks, salts, foams, and teas, to sugar scrubs and natural sun protection and aromatic, deodorizing body powders. The end-products are so delightfully soothing and pampering that you'll want to lavish as much attention on your body as possible. Remember: *Pampering* is not a dirty word; it's a downright necessity!

Cultivating good body care habits not only improves your exterior appearance and prolongs youthful radiance, but also enhances how you feel about yourself, giving you an air of confidence and a healthy dose of self-esteem.

Note that many of the recipes in this book and in this section perform double duty and can be used for the body as well as the face, as the application tips in individual recipes indicate.

Body Moisturizers: Creams, Butters, and Balms

All moisturizers, whether rich and heavy or light and silky, act to improve the skin's barrier function by locking and sealing moisture in and preventing evaporation. Applying moisturizer is a *daily essential,* a vitally important skin care step that should never be skipped.

SESAME AND SHEA BUTTERY BODY OIL

*I*n addition to being one of the best all-over skin softeners, this blend is excellent as a spot treatment for dry heels, knees, and elbows and makes a perfect nightly cuticle conditioning oil. Men also enjoy this thick oil with its warm, softly spicy, stimulating scent.

5 tablespoons sesame base oil

3 tablespoons shea butter, refined or unrefined

10 drops **each** of the following essential oils: cardamom; ginger; sweet orange

RECOMMENDED FOR: *all skin types except oily and combination*
USE: *daily or as desired*
PREP TIME: *approximately 20 minutes, plus 24 hours to completely thicken*
BLENDING TOOLS: *small whisk or spoon*
STORE IN: *plastic squeeze bottle*
YIELD: *½ cup*

In a small saucepan over low heat or in a double boiler, warm the sesame oil and shea butter until the shea butter is just melted. Remove from heat and gently stir for 1 minute to blend ingredients, then allow the mixture to cool to body temperature. Add the essential oils and stir again.

Pour into a storage container.

Note: Unlike beeswax, shea butter takes a long time to completely thicken. This formula will need about 24 hours to completely set up. When it's ready, it will be thick and a pale, creamy yellow color.

No refrigeration is required, but for maximum freshness and potency, please use within 6 to 12 months.

APPLICATION TIPS: Immediately following a bath or shower, while your skin is still damp, slather this oil blend on your body — really massage it in. Because it's very concentrated, begin with 1 teaspoon at a time.

PROTECTION CREAM

*I*n *the cooler months I use this cream all over my body, especially on areas that need extra attention, such as rough shins, knees, hands, and feet, and I often slather it on right before bedtime. An added bonus: It smells subtly of tropical suntan lotion.*

1	tablespoon cocoa butter
2	tablespoons beeswax
¼	cup coconut base oil (extra-virgin; unrefined)
½	cup plus 1 tablespoon almond, soybean, or apricot kernel base oil

RECOMMENDED FOR: *all skin types (but don't use on areas that are exceptionally oily or blemished)*
USE: *daily or as desired*
PREP TIME: *approximately 20 to 30 minutes, plus overnight to completely set*
BLENDING TOOLS: *small whisk or spoon*
STORE IN: *plastic or glass jar or tin*
YIELD: *approximately 1 cup*

In a small saucepan over low heat or in a double boiler, warm all ingredients until the coconut oil, beeswax, and cocoa butter are just melted.

Remove from heat and allow the mixture to cool for 5 to 10 minutes, then gently stir with small whisk or spoon for about 1 minute. Allow it to cool and thicken a bit more, then continue stirring until the mixture is opaque but pourable. (Setting the pan in a shallow ice-water bath speeds the process.)

Pour the cream into storage container(s) and cap. Let it set overnight to give the cocoa butter plenty of time to completely harden.

Note: If the temperature is above 76°F, the cream will maintain a softer consistency. (Coconut oil turns from solid to liquid at 76°F.) If the temperature is below 76°F, the cream will be firmer. If it's too firm for your liking, set the storage container in a shallow pan of hot water for 5 to 10 minutes before use.

No refrigeration is required, but for maximum freshness and potency, please use within 6 to 12 months.

APPLICATION TIPS: Immediately following a bath or shower, while your skin is still damp, slather your body with this cream. Because it's very concentrated, begin with 1 teaspoon at a time. If skin has an oily residue after 5 minutes, you've used too much. Simply wipe off the excess with a coarse towel.

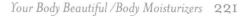

Baby's Bottom Cream

I originally created this cream for infants and small children to protect against diaper rash and soothe occasional bouts of dermatitis, but I've discovered that it also makes a great "ski cream" or barrier cream when your skin is exposed to cold, dry, air or cold, windy weather. It also makes a great cuticle cream and moisturizes cracked heels, elbows, and rough knees.

2 tablespoons almond, soybean, sesame, extra-virgin olive, or macadamia nut base oil	RECOMMENDED FOR: *all skin types in need of protection from the elements, especially dry or rashy skin*
2 tablespoons nonpetroleum jelly	USE: *as desired*
1 tablespoon cocoa butter	PREP TIME: *approximately 20 minutes, plus overnight to completely set*
1 teaspoon beeswax	BLENDING TOOLS: *small whisk or spoon*
2 drops calendula (CO$_2$ extract), Roman chamomile, sweet orange, or rose otto essential oil	STORE IN: *plastic or glass jar*
	YIELD: *approximately 5 tablespoons or ⅓ cup*

In a small saucepan over low heat or in a double boiler, warm all ingredients except the essential oil until the wax and cocoa butter are just melted.

Remove from heat and stir with small whisk or spoon for about 1 minute, then allow the mixture to cool until it becomes slightly opaque. Add the essential oil and stir again to remove any lumps.

Pour into storage container(s) and cap. Allow it to set overnight to give the cocoa butter plenty of time to completely harden. No refrigeration is required, but for maximum freshness and potency, please use within 6 to 12 months.

APPLICATION TIPS: A little goes a long way, so be judicious with the quantity you apply. This cream can be applied anywhere there is dry skin or where moisture needs to be sealed in and dehydrating air sealed out. Think of it as a natural version of petroleum jelly.

CRAZY FOR COCONUT BALM

This product smells luscious, tastes delicious (it's safe to taste), and is simple to make. Many people swear by coconut oil's ability to melt right into the skin and use it from head to toe year-round as a superb body beautifier.

7 tablespoons coconut base oil (extra-virgin, unrefined)

1 tablespoon cocoa butter

40 drops vanilla or sweet orange essential oil (optional)

RECOMMENDED FOR: *all skin types except oily and combination*
USE: *daily or as desired*
PREP TIME: *approximately 20 minutes, plus 2 hours to solidify if weather is cool*
BLENDING TOOLS: *small spoon*
STORE IN: *plastic or glass jar if weather is cool; plastic squeeze bottle if temperature is above 76°F*
YIELD: *approximately ½ cup*

In a small pan over low heat or in a double boiler, warm coconut oil and cocoa butter until the butter is just melted. Remove from heat and let cool for 15 minutes. Add the essential oil and stir to blend. Pour into storage container(s) and cap. Allow the mixture to set for 2 hours.

Note: If the temperature of your storage area is above 76°F, the balm will maintain a liquid consistency. (Coconut oil turns from solid to liquid at 76°F.) If the temperature is below 76°F, the balm will be firm. Remember, too, that coconut oil and cocoa butter will melt on contact with skin.

No refrigeration is required, but for maximum freshness and potency, please use within 1 year.

APPLICATION TIPS: Immediately following a bath or shower, while your skin is still damp, slather this oil blend on your body — really massage it in. Because it's very concentrated, begin with 1 teaspoon at a time.

Blue Chamomile and Olive Body Butter

*T*his herbal butter deeply feeds your skin from the outside. It makes a fabulous cleansing cream and facial moisturizer for all skin types and a wonderful nail conditioning cream. It even works well as an antifrizz hair conditioner if applied sparingly to the ends of dry, fine, frizzy hair, and is a great anti-inflammatory after-sun cream. For the chamomile-infused oil, either make your own (see Oil of Sunshine: The Ultimate Herbal Comfort Oil on page 338 for instructions) or purchase it from a health-food store or mail-order supplier.

¾ cup extra-virgin olive base oil or chamomile-infused olive oil

⅓ cup coconut base oil (must be extra-virgin and unrefined)

4 tablespoons beeswax

2 teaspoons anhydrous lanolin

1 cup distilled water or rosemary, chamomile, or lavender hydrosol

30 drops German chamomile essential oil

30 drops Roman chamomile essential oil

RECOMMENDED FOR: *all skin types especially inflamed, irritated skin*
USE: *daily*
PREP TIME: *approximately 20 to 30 minutes, plus 30 minutes to completely cool and set*
BLENDING TOOLS: *blender; long, slender spatula*
STORE IN: *plastic or glass jars; it's especially beautiful in cobalt blue or dark green glass*
YIELD: *approximately 2⅓ cups*

HEAT: In a saucepan over low heat or in a double boiler, warm the base oils, beeswax, and lanolin until the wax is just melted. In another pan, warm the water or hydrosol.

COOL: Remove both pans from heat and allow their contents to cool almost to body temperature, until the oils/wax/lanolin mixture just begins to thicken and becomes slightly opaque. It should be the consistency of a soft, loose salve. This will take approximately 5 to 10 minutes, depending on the temperature of your kitchen. As it thickens, give the mixture a few stirs to remove any lumps.

BLEND: Immediately pour the mixture into the blender, scraping the sides of the pan to remove every last trace. Place the lid on the blender and remove the lid's plastic piece. Turn the blender on medium and slowly drizzle the water or hydrosol through the center of the lid into the vortex of swirling fats below. Closely watch what happens: Almost immediately, the body butter will begin to thicken. Blend for 5 to 10 seconds more, turn off the blender, and check the consistency of the butter. It should have a smooth texture. If the water isn't combining thoroughly with the fat mixture, turn off the blender and give the mixture a few stirs with a spatula to free up the blender blades. Then replace the lid and blend on medium to high for another 10 seconds. Repeat as necessary. The body butter will be thick.

Turn off the blender and add the essential oils, manually stirring a few times to incorporate them, then blend completely on medium for another 5 to 10 seconds.

Note: If the temperature of your kitchen is above 76°F, the body butter will maintain a softer consistency. If the temperature is below 76°F, the body butter will be firmer.

PACKAGE AND COOL: Spoon the finished body butter into storage container(s). Lightly cover each container with a paper towel and allow the blend to cool for 30 minutes before capping. If you notice, after a few hours or days, that water begins to separate from your body butter, don't worry. The mixture can separate if the fat temperature and water temperature are not relatively equal and cool enough when the two portions are blended. Keep trying — making perfect creams is an art!

No refrigeration is required if used within 30 days. If refrigerated, please use within 3 to 6 months. (Refrigeration may change the texture of the product, but potency will not be affected.)

APPLICATION TIPS: Immediately following a bath or shower, slather this butter on your damp skin — really massage it in. Because it's very concentrated, begin with 1 teaspoon at a time. If skin has an oily residue after 5 minutes, you've used too much. Simply wipe off the excess with a coarse towel and use less the next time around.

Bath Therapy: The Aromatic and "Scentual" Bath

Bathing has been a revered ritual for thousands of years. Cleopatra was known for taking soothing milk baths; Marie Antoinette for taking long, luxurious herbal soaks; the Romans for enjoying public, social baths; and the North American Indians for their purifying sweat lodge experience followed by a quick plunge into a cold stream or river.

A bath is a wonderful way to pamper, soothe, rejuvenate, and refresh the senses. Taking a bath can also create some much-needed private time to luxuriate in skin conditioning waters.

Healing treatments can be incorporated into the bathing ritual, too. Health spas the world over offer mineral baths in hot springs, sulfur waters, and clay (used to remove impurities from the skin). Various herbal and salt baths are also enjoyable for their fragrant, soothing, and therapeutic benefits.

Whether you're interested in soaking away your tired, aching muscles and daily tensions; stimulating your circulation; softening your dry skin; or enjoying calming waters laced with lavender, rose, or chamomile essential oil; these recipes are sure to please. Shower fanatics beware: Try a few of these tub-tantalizing mixtures and you may become a true bath lover after all!

Note: Please keep bath water warm, not hot, unless otherwise indicated in the recipe. The hotter the water, the quicker the volatile essential oils dissipate into the air and lose their healing qualities. Hot water also dehydrates your skin — and that's not the desired result of all this bathing bliss!

BASIC HERBAL BATH BAG

This bag has the perfect combination of herbs and oats to soothe even the most sensitive skin.

1   9- by 9-inch square of muslin or cheesecloth, or toe of a nylon stocking

2   tablespoons elder flowers, chamomile flowers, lavender buds, or lemon balm leaves

2   tablespoons comfrey leaves

2   tablespoons ground oatmeal

1   tablespoon blackberry leaves

String or yarn

RECOMMENDED FOR: *all skin types, especially itchy or rashy skin*
USE: *as desired*
FOLLOW WITH: *moisturizer*
PREP TIME: *approximately 10 minutes (if oatmeal is ground ahead of time)*
STORE IN: *zip-seal plastic bag, plastic or glass jar, or tin (if making several bags at once)*
YIELD: *1 treatment*

Place ingredients in the center of the cloth or the toe of the stocking. Gather the material into a loose pouch and tie with a string or yarn long enough to hang from the hot water tap in the tub (the running water will flow through the bag).

No refrigeration is required for extra bags, but store in a dry, airtight container, and for maximum freshness and potency, please use within 6 months.

APPLICATION TIPS: After hanging the bag and filling the tub, untie the bag and let it float in the water. Sit back and enjoy! Soak for 20 to 30 minutes. Discard the bag when finished.

Skin Softening Wash Bag

T his bag does wonders for dry, itchy, scaly skin and skin suffering from any poison plant rash or general dermatitis.

1   9- by 9-inch square of muslin or cheesecloth, or toe of a nylon stocking

¼   cup ground oatmeal

¼   cup ground sunflower seeds

String or yarn

RECOMMENDED FOR: *all skin types, especially dry and sensitive*
USE: *as desired*
FOLLOW WITH: *moisturizer*
PREP TIME: *approximately 10 minutes (if meals are ground ahead of time)*
STORE IN: *zip-seal plastic bag, plastic or glass jar, or tin (if making several bags at once)*
YIELD: *1 treatment*

Place ingredients in the center of the cloth or the toe of the stocking. Gather the material into a loose pouch and tie with a short string or yarn.

No refrigeration is required for extra bags, but store in a dry, airtight container, and for maximum freshness and potency, please use within 6 months.

APPLICATION TIPS: When ready to bathe, toss the bag into the water as the tub fills. As you relax in the tub for 20 to 30 minutes, gently rub your entire body with the bag, then let it remain in the water, where it can continue to release its skin-softening properties. Discard the bag when finished.

STIMULATING HERBAL BATH BAG

This bag is the perfect pick-me-up to use prior to going out for a night on the town. It stimulates the circulation and enlivens the senses while softening the skin.

1   9- by 9-inch square of muslin or cheesecloth, or toe of a nylon stocking

2   tablespoons peppermint leaves

2   tablespoons rosemary leaves

1   tablespoon basil leaves

1   tablespoon dried (or 2 tablespoons fresh) finely chopped lemon rind

1   tablespoon dried (or 2 tablespoons fresh) finely chopped orange rind

1   tablespoon ground oatmeal or sunflower seed meal

5   drops peppermint essential oil

5   drops rosemary (chemotype verbenon) essential oil

String or yarn

RECOMMENDED FOR: *all skin types except sensitive, sunburned, or windburned skin*
USE: *as desired*
FOLLOW WITH: *moisturizer*
PREP TIME: *approximately 15 minutes (if meal is ground ahead of time)*
STORE IN: *zip-seal plastic bag, plastic or glass jar, or tin (if making several bags at once)*
YIELD: *1 treatment*

Place dry ingredients in the center of the cloth or the toe of the stocking. Add essential oils to the mix. Gather the material into a loose pouch and tie with a string or yarn long enough to hang from the hot water tap in the tub (the running water will flow through the bag).

No refrigeration is required for extra bags, but store in a dry, air-tight container, and for maximum freshness and potency, please use within 6 months. *Note:* If you're making extra bags to store, use only dried orange and lemon rind. (The fresh versions will mold.)

APPLICATION TIPS: After hanging the bag filling the tub, untie the bag and let it float in the water. Relax in the tub for 20 to 30 minutes, gently rubbing your entire body with the bag. Discard the bag when finished.

Garden of Flowers Relaxing Bath Bag

This bath bag was created for the flower gardener in all of us. There's nothing quite like bathing in a tub of floral fragrance. This is soothing to the psyche as well as the skin.

1   9- by 9-inch square of muslin or cheesecloth, or toe of a nylon stocking

2   tablespoons calendula blossoms

2   tablespoons chamomile flowers

2   tablespoons lavender buds

2   tablespoons rose petals (or, in place of the these flowers, blossoms, and buds, use 4 tablespoons fresh chamomile flowers and 4 tablespoons fresh lavender buds or rose petals)

1   tablespoon ground oatmeal or sunflower seed meal

10 drops Roman chamomile or 5 drops lavender and 5 drops rose otto essential oil

String or yarn

RECOMMENDED FOR: *all skin types, especially sensitive skin*
USE: *as desired*
FOLLOW WITH: *moisturizer*
PREP TIME: *approximately 15 minutes (if meal is ground ahead of time)*
STORE IN: *zip-seal plastic bag, plastic or glass jar, or tin (if making several bags at once)*
YIELD: *1 treatment*

Place dry ingredients in the center of the cloth or the toe of the stocking. Add essential oils to the mix. Gather the material into a loose pouch and tie with a string or yarn long enough to hang from the hot water tap in the tub (the running water will flow through the bag).

No refrigeration is required for extra bags, but store in a dry, air-tight container, and for maximum freshness and potency, please use within 6 months. *Note:* If you're making extra bags to store, use only dried flowers. (The fresh versions will mold.)

APPLICATION TIPS: After hanging the bag and filling the tub, untie the bag and let it float in the water. As you relax in the tub for 20 to 30 minutes, gently rub your entire body with the bag. Discard the bag when finished.

Basic Milk Bath

This makes a wonderful soak for itchy, rashy, or weather-beaten dry skin. It leaves skin feeling silky soft.

½ cup powdered whole or nonfat milk

1 tablespoon apricot kernel, jojoba, sunflower, or favorite base oil

10 drops Roman chamomile, lavender, geranium, or rosemary (chemotype *verbenon*) essential oil (optional)

RECOMMENDED FOR: *all skin types (if skin is oily, omit oil from recipe)*
USE: *as desired*
FOLLOW WITH: *moisturizer*
PREP TIME: *approximately 5 minutes*
STORE IN: *do not store; mix as needed*
YIELD: *1 treatment*

Pour the powdered milk and the base oil together directly under running bath water. Add the essential oil (if desired) immediately before stepping into tub. Swish the water with your hands to mix.

APPLICATION TIPS: Relax. Submerse your entire body in this moisturizing bath for 20 to 30 minutes.

FLOWERS AND SPICE STRESS-RELIEVING MILKY BATH SALTS

T*his is a warming, calming, de-stressing bath blend for the high-strung person who has a tendency to feel chilled all the time. It helps relieve muscle aches while simultaneously softening the skin.*

½ cup Epsom salt

½ cup powdered whole
    or nonfat milk

2   drops **each** of the following
    essential oils: vanilla; rose
    otto or geranium; cardamom

RECOMMENDED FOR: *all skin types*
USE: *as desired*
FOLLOW WITH: *moisturizer*
PREP TIME: *approximately 5 minutes*
STORE IN: *do not store; mix as needed*
YIELD: *1 treatment*

Pour the Epsom salt and the powdered milk together directly under running bath water. Add the essential oils immediately before stepping into tub. Swish the water with your hands to mix.

No refrigeration is required if you make an extra batch or two, but store salts in a dry, airtight container, and for maximum freshness and potency, please use within 6 months.

APPLICATION TIPS: Relax. Soak for 20 to 30 minutes.

Ginger and Orange Stimulating Milky Bath Salts

This bag provides a stimulating, warming, slightly spicy bath blend. It helps relieve lethargy and muscle aches while simultaneously softening the skin.

1   10- by 10-inch square of muslin or cheesecloth or toe of a nylon stocking

½   cup Epsom salt

½   cup powdered whole or nonfat milk

1   tablespoon dried (or 2 tablespoons fresh) finely chopped orange rind

1   tablespoon powdered dried ginger

1   tablespoon rosemary leaves

5   drops ginger essential oil

5   drops sweet orange essential oil

String or yarn

RECOMMENDED FOR: *all skin types except sensitive*
USE: *as desired*
FOLLOW WITH: *moisturizer*
PREP TIME: *approximately 15 minutes*
STORE IN: *zip-seal plastic bag, plastic or glass jar, or tin (if making several bags at once)*
YIELD: *1 treatment*

Place dry ingredients in the center of the cloth or the toe of the stocking. Add essential oils to the mix. Gather the material into a loose pouch and tie with a string or yarn long enough to hang from the hot water tap in the tub (the running water will flow through the bag).

No refrigeration is required if you make an extra batch or two, but store salts in a dry, airtight container, and for maximum freshness and potency, please use within 6 months. *Note:* If you're making an extra bags to store, use only dried orange rind. (The fresh version will mold.)

APPLICATION TIPS: After hanging the bag and filling the tub, untie the bag and let it float in the water. Soak for 20 to 30 minutes. Discard the bag when finished.

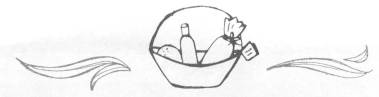

Bath Therapy Gift Idea

Bath salts are an easy-to-make, inexpensive, and warmly welcomed gift.

- Whip up a large batch of the Simple Herbal Bath Salts (page 235) — enough for about four baths.
- Find a decorative tin or jar with a tight-fitting lid and fill it with the bath salts. (To absorb any moisture that might find its way into the container, put a small muslin or mesh bag of rice in the bottom.)
- Tie a piece of ribbon or twine around the container and attach a small wooden or scallop-shell scoop and a hand-printed card detailing instructions for use.

This great gift will give plenty of relaxation and pleasure to a stress-weary relative or friend.

HONEY CREAM BATH

This is an ultra-pampering, luxurious, hydrating bath blend formulated to moisturize the driest of skin. The combination of emollient cream with soothing, healing, humectant honey feels great on parched, irritated skin.

1 cup heavy cream or half-and-half

½ cup raw honey at room temperature

RECOMMENDED FOR: *all skin types, especially dry, dehydrated, environmentally damaged, sunburned, or windburned skin*
USE: *as desired*
FOLLOW WITH: *moisturizer*
PREP TIME: *approximately 5 minutes*
STORE IN: *do not store; mix as needed*
YIELD: *1 treatment*

Pour the cream and the honey together directly under running bath water. Swish the water with your hands to mix before getting into the tub.

APPLICATION TIPS: Relax. Submerse your entire body for 20 to 30 minutes.

SIMPLE HERBAL BATH SALTS

This bath softens, soothes, and heals rough, irritated skin while the natural essential oil (whichever one you choose) calms the mind and body, preparing you for sleep. It's best to take this bath right before sliding between the sheets.

½ cup baking soda

½ cup sea salt

15 drops calendula (CO2 extract), lavender, or Roman chamomile essential oil

RECOMMENDED FOR: *all skin types, especially itchy, rashy skin (avoid if skin is abraded or highly sensitive)*
USE: *as desired*
FOLLOW WITH: *moisturizer*
PREP TIME: *approximately 5 minutes*
STORE IN: *zip-seal plastic bag, plastic or glass jar, or tin (if making a larger amount of bath salts)*
YIELD: *1 treatment*

Turn on the tap full blast and pour the soda and the salt into the tub. When the tub is full, add the essential oil and swish the water with your hands to mix.

No refrigeration is required if you make an extra batch or two, but store salts in a dry, airtight container, and for maximum freshness and potency, please use within 6 months.

APPLICATION TIPS: Soak for 20 to 30 minutes.

LAVENDER LOVER'S BATH SALTS

For the lavender lover, there's nothing like a relaxing, skin-pampering, healing bath heavily fragranced with old-fashioned lavender. The aroma escorts your senses to the lavender fields of France. This bath blend is good for a tired, achy body, especially if the joints are swollen and the muscles are strained from overuse. It's best to take this bath right before going to bed. Follow it with a head-to-toe slathering of a therapeutic lavender body cream or massage oil, then slip into your favorite flannel pajamas and don thick socks. You'll sleep like a baby!

1	10- by 10-inch square of muslin or cheesecloth, or toe of a nylon stocking
1	cup lavender buds
20	drops lavender essential oil
	String or yarn
1	cup Epsom salt
½	cup baking soda

RECOMMENDED FOR: *all skin types, especially irritated or inflamed skin (avoid if skin is abraded or highly sensitive)*
USE: *as desired*
FOLLOW WITH: *moisturizer*
PREP TIME: *approximately 15 minutes*
STORE IN: *zip-seal plastic bag, plastic or glass jar, or tin (if making several bags at once)*
YIELD: *1 treatment*

Place the lavender buds in the center of the cloth or the toe of the stocking. Add the essential oil by the drop to the buds. Gather the material into a loose pouch and tie with a string or yarn long enough to hang from the hot water tap in the tub (the running water will flow through the bag). Pour the salt and baking soda directly under the running bath water to dissolve.

No refrigeration is required if you make an extra batch or two, but store salts in a dry, airtight container, and for maximum freshness and potency, please use within 6 months.

APPLICATION TIPS: After hanging the bag and filling the tub, untie the bag and let it float in the water. Gently exfoliate and fragrance the skin by massaging your entire body with the lavender bag. Discard the bag when finished.

SORE MUSCLE SOAK

This bath helps relax tense, sore muscles yet doesn't leave you smelling of a medicinal vapor rub. The aroma will soothe frayed nerves but won't lull you to sleep.

1   12- by 12-inch square of
    muslin or cheesecloth, or
    toe of a nylon stocking
1   cup Epsom salt
½   cup baking soda
1   tablespoon chamomile flowers
1   tablespoon juniper berries
1   tablespoon pine needles
1   tablespoon sage leaves
2   teaspoons lemon balm leaves
2   teaspoons peppermint leaves
15 drops eucalyptus, peppermint,
    or juniper essential oil
String or yarn

RECOMMENDED FOR: *all skin types except abraded or highly sensitive*
USE: *following exercise, or as desired*
FOLLOW WITH: *moisturizer*
PREP TIME: *approximately 15 minutes*
STORE IN: *zip-seal plastic bag, plastic or glass jar, or tin (if making several bags at once)*
YIELD: *1 treatment*

Place dry ingredients in the center of the cloth or the toe of the stocking. Add the essential oils to the mix. Gather the material into a loose pouch and tie with a string or yarn long enough to hang from the hot water tap in the tub (the running water will flow through the bag).

No refrigeration is required if you make an extra batch or two, but store salts in a dry, airtight container, and for maximum freshness and potency, please use within 6 months.

APPLICATION TIPS: After hanging the bag and filling the tub, untie the bag and let it float in the water. Soak for 20 to 30 minutes. Discard the bag when finished.

Vinegar Bath

*T*his bath soothes and softens itchy skin, relieves the sting of sunburn and wind-burn, and reestablishes proper skin pH levels. It also makes a good deodorizing foot bath additive.

4   cups apple cider vinegar
    (does not have to be raw)

½   cup rosemary leaves or
    juniper berries (Either herb
    may be halved in quantity
    and mixed with comfrey root
    to create a mucilaginous,
    comforting blend.)

RECOMMENDED FOR: *all skin types except abraded or very sensitive*
USE: *as desired*
FOLLOW WITH: *moisturizer*
PREP TIME: *3 to 4 hours*
BLENDING TOOLS: *strainer*
STORE IN: *decorative glass bottle or any glass container*
YIELD: *approximately 4 cups*

In a medium-sized saucepan, bring the vinegar to just shy of boiling. Remove from heat and add the herbs. Cover and allow to steep for 3 to 4 hours. Strain and store in a pretty container.

No refrigeration is required, but for maximum freshness and potency, please use within 1 year.

APPLICATION TIPS: Add 1 cup to bath while tap is running. Soak 20 to 30 minutes.

HERBAL ANTICELLULITE DETOX BATH TEA

*T*his bath is designed to help relieve water retention. Cellulite results from accumulated toxins and water trapped in subsurface skin tissues. The result: that lumpy, spongy texture. The herbs in this blend act as circulatory stimulants and diuretics.

1	gallon purified water
1	cup dried chopped ginger root (or 2 cups fresh)
½	cup juniper berries
½	cup rosemary leaves
½	cup thyme leaves
1	cup Epsom salt
10	drops geranium essential oil
5	drops juniper essential oil
3	drops cedarwood essential oil
3	drops grapefruit essential oil

RECOMMENDED FOR: *all skin types with cellulite except sensitive skin (avoid bath entirely if you have a history of kidney problems)*
USE: *2 times per week*
FOLLOW WITH: *moisturizer*
PREP TIME: *approximately 3 to 4 hours*
BLENDING TOOLS: *large strainer*
STORE IN: *do not store; mix as needed*
YIELD: *1 treatment*

In a large pan, bring the water to a boil. Remove from heat and add the herbs. Cover and steep for 3 to 4 hours, then strain, squeezing infusion from herbs. Turn on the bath tap full blast (the water temperature should be quite warm) and pour in the Epsom salt and the herbal infusion. Add the essential oils and swish the water with your hands to blend. (It's important that the essential oils are well blended with the water and other ingredients before you step into the tub.)

APPLICATION TIPS: To aid the herb's penetration into the skin, dry brush your entire body before bathing. (See directions on page 36.) While soaking for 20 to 30 minutes, drink 2 full glasses of hot, purified water laced with 2 teaspoons of fresh lemon juice. It's important to sweat during this bath. The water, lemon, and sweating action flush toxins from the body via the kidneys and perspiration. Following the bath, dry off with a coarse towel, concentrating your efforts on areas with cellulite.

Bubblicious Herbal Bath Foam

This is an easy-to-make alternative to chemical-laden commercial foaming bath products. The recipe doubles as a hair shampoo, face cleanser, or body wash and makes a great travel product! Note that natural foaming agents do not produce quite as many suds as commercial products.

1   8-ounce bottle natural shampoo base, unscented

40   drops favorite essential oil such as lavender, ginger, Roman chamomile, spearmint, geranium, grapefruit, rose otto, vanilla, or ylang ylang

RECOMMENDED FOR: *all skin types except dry or dehydrated skin*
USE: *as desired*
FOLLOW WITH: *moisturizer*
PREP TIME: *approximately 5 minutes*
BLENDING TOOLS: *shake bottle prior to use*
STORE IN: *shampoo base bottle or decorative bottle of choice*
YIELD: *1 cup or 8 ounces*

Add the essential oil to the bottle of shampoo base and shake well to blend.

No refrigeration is required, but for maximum freshness and potency, please use within 1 year.

APPLICATION TIPS: Turn on the tap full blast and pour ¼ cup of bath foam into the tub. Soak for 20 to 30 minutes.

Bath and Massage Oils

Bath and massage oils (or body oils) are easy to make at home and act as lubricants and emollient moisture barriers that help to keep skin hydrated following a bath or shower. Applied during a high-friction massage, a body oil is readily absorbed, penetrating skin tissues and supplying therapeutic skin conditioning.

My favorite body oil base is jojoba, as it does not need refrigeration, will not go rancid, and is chemically quite similar to human sebum, but lighter oils such as apricot, almond, sunflower, hazelnut, soybean, and macadamia nut work just as well (though they must be refrigerated). Sesame, avocado, and extra-virgin olive oil are heavy and can have quite a distinctive aroma that some may dislike. Sesame oil, though, can impart a velvety texture to the skin that I love — especially in midwinter, when my skin is driest. Unrefined coconut oil is a favorite body oil base for many who enjoy the exquisite fragrance.

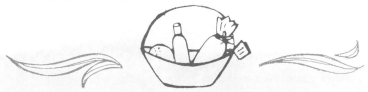

Bath and Massage Oil Gift Idea

- Bath oils make the perfect gift for a friend who has a stressful lifestyle and enjoys unwinding with a long, luxurious bath.
- Massage oils (and an accompanying massage gift certificate to a local spa) are a great treat for a special friend.
- Package your gift oil in a decorative blue, green, or brown glass bottle to protect the essential oils and base oils from exposure to light. Make sure the bottle you use is sterilized and has a tight-fitting lid!
- Create a custom label for your bottle and attach a gift card with your personalized message and simple directions for use.

Velvety Vanilla Oil

This oil has a relaxing vanilla aroma and easily melts into the skin, leaving no oily residue. It's ideal to use during a partner massage or as a full-body moisturizing perfume. I use this oil as a scented base oil when making vanilla creams and lotions.

3   long (6- or 7-inch) vanilla
    beans
    (or substitute 100 drops
    vanilla essential oil)
1 ½ cups jojoba base oil

RECOMMENDED FOR: *all skin types, even oily*
USE: *as desired*
FOLLOW WITH: *moisturize body after bath or shower if necessary*
PREP TIME: *approximately 10 minutes, plus 2 months to complete infusion*
BLENDING TOOLS: *glass jar; strainer, coffee filter, or nylon stocking; shake bottle prior to use*
STORE IN: *glass bottle or plastic squeeze bottle*
YIELD: *approximately 1½ cups*

Slice the vanilla beans lengthwise, scrape out paste from each pod, and add it to a pint-size or smaller glass jar. Chop the empty bean pods into 1-inch pieces and add to the jar. Pour in the base oil. (Add the essential oil now if vanilla beans are unavailable.) Cap the jar and shake the mixture for 1 minute.

Store the jar in a dark place for 2 months to allow the vanilla essence to infuse the oil. During this time, shake the jar every day for 10 to 15 seconds.

After 2 months, strain the oil through a tight-mesh strainer, coffee filter, or nylon stocking, then pour the oil into an elegant glass storage bottle (though a plastic squeeze bottle is more convenient for use). The finished oil will have a deep, round vanilla fragrance.

Note: Jojoba base oil will harden in a cold area. To soften it, simply leave it at room temperature for an hour or set the bottle in a shallow pan of hot water for 10 minutes.

No refrigeration is required, but for maximum fragrance, please use within 2 years.

APPLICATION TIPS: For bath oil, add 2 teaspoons to running water. Use as needed for a body or massage oil.

NOURISHING OIL

This is a nourishing blend that's high in essential fatty acids. It doubles as a healing oil to massage into cuticles on a nightly basis, especially if the cuticles are dry and ragged. It helps promote nail growth and a natural sheen on the nail surface.

3   tablespoons sesame seed base oil
1   tablespoon **each** of the following base oils: almond, extra-virgin olive, avocado, macadamia nut, and apricot kernel
2   large vitamin E oil capsules

RECOMMENDED FOR: *all skin types, including oily*
USE: *as desired*
FOLLOW WITH: *moisturize body after bath or shower if necessary*
PREP TIME: *approximately 10 minutes*
BLENDING TOOLS: *shake bottle prior to use*
STORE IN: *glass bottle or plastic squeeze bottle*
YIELD: *approximately ½ cup*

Combine all ingredients in a storage bottle. Tightly cap the bottle and shake the mixture vigorously.

No refrigeration is required if product is to be used within 6 months. Store in the refrigerator for up to 1 year.

APPLICATION TIPS: For bath oil, add 2 teaspoons to running water. For application as a body oil following a shower or for massage, use as needed.

FLORAL OIL

This is an especially fragrant, romantic blend reminiscent of a spring garden. It's deeply conditioning to skin while simultaneously balancing sebum production. Women and little girls love this oil! It makes a wonderful after-bath oil for infant girls — it leaves them smelling delicately sweet and feminine.

To make a glorious floral perfume, mix the essential oils with 1 tablespoon jojoba base oil and store in a beautiful, tiny glass bottle. Cap the bottle tightly and shake well. Whenever you like, apply just a touch to your pulse points: the base of the neck, wrists, sternum, and behind the knees.

1 cup jojoba base oil
20 drops **each** of the following essential oils: rose otto; lavender; geranium; ylang ylang

RECOMMENDED FOR: *all skin types, including oily*
USE: *as desired*
FOLLOW WITH: *moisturize body after bath or shower if necessary*
PREP TIME: *approximately 10 minutes*
BLENDING TOOLS: *shake bottle prior to use*
STORE IN: *glass bottle or plastic squeeze bottle*
YIELD: *approximately 1 cup*

Combine all ingredients in a storage bottle. Tightly cap the bottle and shake the mixture vigorously.

Note: If your storage area is cold, jojoba oil will harden. To soften it before use, simply leave it at room temperature for an hour or so or set the bottle in a shallow pan of hot water for 10 minutes.

No refrigeration is required, but for maximum fragrance and potency, please use within 2 years.

APPLICATION TIPS: For bath oil, add 2 teaspoons to running water. For application as a body oil following a shower or for massage, use as needed.

Stimulating Herbal Oil

This makes an invigorating, skin-conditioning oil blend. It's great to use after your morning shower — it really enlivens the senses. If you use basil and rosemary essential oils (40 drops of each) in your formula, this particular recipe can double as a scalp-stimulating, hair-growth formula.

1   cup jojoba base oil
80 drops of any one or
    a combination of the
    following essential oils:
    basil, eucalyptus radiata,
    juniper, geranium,
    sweet orange, lemon,
    grapefruit, peppermint,
    spearmint, rosemary,
    and tangerine

RECOMMENDED FOR: *all skin types except sensitive skin*
USE: *as desired*
FOLLOW WITH: *moisturize body after bath or shower if necessary*
PREP TIME: *approximately 10 minutes*
BLENDING TOOLS: *shake bottle prior to use*
STORE IN: *glass bottle or plastic squeeze bottle*
YIELD: *approximately 1 cup*

Combine all ingredients in a storage bottle. Tightly cap the bottle and shake the mixture vigorously.

Note: If your storage area is cold, jojoba oil will harden. To soften it before use, simply leave it at room temperature for an hour or so or set the bottle in a shallow pan of hot water for 10 minutes.

No refrigeration is required, but for maximum fragrance and potency, please use within 2 years.

APPLICATION TIPS: For bath oil, add 2 teaspoons to running water. For application as a body oil following a shower or for massage, use as needed.

TO USE AS A HAIR-GROWTH FORMULA: Simply massage 1 or 2 teaspoons of the blend into dry scalp for 5 minutes; wrap hair in a warm, damp towel; and leave on for 30 minutes. Follow with shampoo and conditioner. Your hair should feel as soft as cat fur!

UPLIFTING COLD AND FLU BATH OIL

I use this oil blend when I'm suffering from a cold or the flu. It helps relieve body aches and unblock sinuses and seems to chase away the mental funk that often accompanies head-to-toe misery. It refreshes and energizes all the senses and doubles as a great deodorizing foot massage oil for tired feet.

3   teaspoons jojoba oil
3   drops **each** of the following essential oils: Roman chamomile, peppermint, rosemary (chemotype verbenon), juniper, and eucalyptus radiata

RECOMMENDED FOR: *all skin types except sensitive*
USE: *as desired*
FOLLOW WITH: *moisturize body after bath if necessary*
PREP TIME: *approximately 5 minutes*
BLENDING TOOLS: *small bowl and spoon*
STORE IN: *do not store; mix as needed*
YIELD: *1 treatment*

Combine all ingredients in a small glass bowl. Stir the mixture vigorously to blend.

APPLICATION TIPS: Add to the bath while the bath water is running.

TO USE AS A FOOT MASSAGE OIL: Simply massage your clean feet (or better yet, have a friend massage them) for 15 minutes, don socks, and go to bed. It really softens tough, scaly skin.

Exotic Oil

This skin conditioning oil warms your body, stimulates circulation, and balances your mood. It's wonderful for weather-beaten and mature skin in need of toning, revitalizing, and renewed suppleness and can also be used as an exotic perfume.

1   cup jojoba base oil
30 drops neroli essential oil
20 drops cardamom essential oil
20 drops ginger essential oil
10 drops frankincense essential oil (CO2 extract)
5   drops clove essential oil

RECOMMENDED FOR: *all skin types except sensitive*
USE: *as desired*
FOLLOW WITH: *moisturize body after bath or shower if necessary*
PREP TIME: *approximately 10 minutes*
BLENDING TOOLS: *shake bottle prior to use*
STORE IN: *glass bottle or plastic squeeze bottle*
YIELD: *approximately 1 cup*

Combine all ingredients in a storage bottle. Tightly cap the bottle and shake the mixture vigorously.

Note: If your storage area is cold, jojoba oil will harden. To soften it before use, simply leave it at room temperature for an hour or so or set the bottle in a shallow pan of hot water for 10 minutes.

No refrigeration is required, but for maximum fragrance and potency, please use within 2 years.

APPLICATION TIPS: For bath oil, add 2 teaspoons to running water. For application as a body oil following a shower or for massage, use as needed.

TO USE AS A PERFUME: Mix the essential oils with 1 tablespoon jojoba base oil and store in a beautiful, tiny glass bottle. Cap the bottle tightly and shake well. Whenever you like, apply just a touch to your pulse points: the base of the neck, wrists, sternum, and behind the knees. Use with caution if skin is sensitive and avoid contact with mucous membranes.

THERAPEUTIC CREAMY MASSAGE BLEND

This blend is designed specifically for sensitive, inflamed, irritated, or bruised skin. It's an anti-inflammatory, skin regenerative oil that acts as a superb wound healer. It also conditions skin that has been overexposed to the elements.

¼ cup plus 2 tablespoons sunflower base oil

¼ cup extra-virgin olive base oil

¼ cup soybean base oil

2 tablespoons shea butter

50 drops helichrysum essential oil

50 drops rosemary (chemotype *verbenon*) essential oil

RECOMMENDED FOR: *all skin types except oily*
USE: *as desired*
FOLLOW WITH: *moisturize body if necessary*
PREP TIME: *approximately 15 minutes, plus 12 hours to thicken*
BLENDING TOOLS: *small whisk or spoon*
STORE IN: *glass bottle or plastic squeeze bottle*
YIELD: *approximately 1 cup*

In a small saucepan, warm the base oils and shea butter over low heat until the shea butter is just melted. Remove from heat and with a small whisk or spoon, briskly stir the mixture for about 15 seconds. Add the essential oils and stir again. Pour the blend into a storage container and cap when almost cool. Because shea butter is slow to thicken, allow up to 12 hours for the product to reach its final, creamy texture.

Note: This creamy, thick oil blend becomes a little bit firmer in cold weather. If you prefer a more liquid consistency, before use simply place the bottle in a pan of hot water for 10 to 20 minutes.

No refrigeration is required, but for maximum freshness and potency, please use within 6 months.

APPLICATION TIPS: Apply as needed to skin immediately after showering or use as a therapeutic creamy massage oil. Shake bottle vigorously prior to each use.

Relaxing Oil

This therapeutic blend has a softly sweet, floral-fruity aroma known to relieve anxiety and calm the nerves. It acts as a muscle relaxant, easing tight, tense muscles and often inducing deep sleep. This oil is the perfect addition to the evening bath or to use during a massage when you have no where to go afterward except to the Land of Nod.

1 cup jojoba base oil
40 drops Roman chamomile essential oil
40 drops ylang ylang essential oil

RECOMMENDED FOR: *all skin types, even oily*
USE: *as desired*
FOLLOW WITH: *moisturize body after bath or shower if necessary*
PREP TIME: *approximately 10 minutes*
BLENDING TOOLS: *shake bottle prior to use*
STORE IN: *glass bottle or plastic squeeze bottle*
YIELD: *approximately 1 cup*

Combine all ingredients in a storage container. Tightly cap the bottle and shake the mixture vigorously.

Note: If storage area is cold, jojoba oil will harden. To soften before use, simply leave at room temperature for an hour or so or set the bottle in a shallow pan of hot water for 10 minutes.

No refrigeration is required, but for maximum fragrance and potency, please use within 2 years.

APPLICATION TIPS: For bath oil, add 2 teaspoons to running water. For application as a body oil following a shower or for massage, use as needed.

Sun Sense: Tanning Potions and After-Sun Relief

In chapter 1, I addressed the health benefits of sun exposure and the importance of appropriate sun protection to prevent potential skin damage (see Step 6: Give Yourself Some Exposure: A Little Sun Is a Good Thing on page 41), but it's important to reiterate that if you want to preserve the beauty and integrity of your skin for years to come and help prevent skin cancer, *do not* spend excessive unprotected time in the sun. Practice holistic sun care: Avoid chemical sunscreens, but do find a natural one that works and offers full-spectrum protection; use common sun sense by staying out of the sun during the high-intensity hours between 10 and 2 or wearing appropriate cover-up clothing; and *always* slather on a good quality, moisturizing lotion or cream, from head to toe to prevent epidermal dehydration.

The natural sun protection recipes that follow have a low SPF of 10 or less and are formulated to nourish and condition your skin before, during, and after exposure to the sun and associated elements such as heat, drying wind, salt water, and chlorine from pools. I've also tossed in a few suggestions for natural remedial action when an unfortunate sunburn does occur. Good advice to remember: As with all things in life, the sun should always be taken in moderation.

SUNSCREEN BODY OIL

The ingredients of this oil combine to form a very hydrating, skin-nourishing blend. If you find yourself suffering from sunburn; windburn; or an itchy rash from sea, sand, salt, or chlorine; this formula is ultra-soothing and aids in healing all irritations.

¼ cup jojoba base oil
¼ cup neem base oil
¼ cup pure aloe vera juice
¼ cup sesame base oil
3 teaspoons vitamin E oil
1 teaspoon anhydrous lanolin

RECOMMENDED FOR: *all skin types except oily*
USE: *before and during sun exposure*
PREP TIME: *approximately 15 minutes*
BLENDING TOOLS: *shake vigorously before each use*
STORE IN: *plastic squeeze bottle*
YIELD: *approximately 1⅛ cup*

Add all ingredients to a storage container. The aloe vera juice is water-based and will separate out (as if you were making an oil and vinegar salad dressing), so the formula must be vigorously shaken each time prior to use.

No refrigeration is required if the product will be used within 3 weeks. If refrigerated, the oil will keep for 4 to 6 months. It will thicken when chilled but will liquefy when allowed to warm to room temperature.

APPLICATION TIPS: Apply to the entire body immediately before and repeatedly during sun exposure. The base oils won't leave an oily film if massaged in thoroughly (unless too much is applied).

A NOTE ABOUT SUNSCREENS

I believe that the best nonchemical, highly effective natural sunscreens on the market today are the sunblocks containing minerals such as micronized titanium dioxide or zinc oxide, which act as physical reflective barriers to the sun (as opposed to potentially toxic, chemical-based sunscreens that actually absorb the suns rays). Most mineral-based sunscreens can be used by those with sensitive skin and they are relatively sweat-proof and waterproof.

Tropical Creamy Body Oil

This oil is designed for the die-hard sun worshipper who tans easily and rarely burns. Its SPF is low but its aroma is oh-so-sweet! It may make you want to bake in the sun all day — but don't! It's highly emollient and beneficial for any part of the body in need of softening.

½ cup coconut base oil (extra-virgin; unrefined)

½ cup jojoba base oil (may substitute sesame or neem oil, but either will produce a warm, ripe, nutty aroma)

2 tablespoons cocoa butter

A few drops coconut fragrance oil (Optional, but smells divine! Follow manufacturer's directions for appropriate amount to add to 1 cup of oil.)

RECOMMENDED FOR: *all skin types except oily*
USE: *before, during, and after sun exposure*
PREP TIME: *approximately 20 minutes, plus 12 hours to thicken*
BLENDING TOOLS: *small spoon or whisk*
STORE IN: *plastic squeeze bottle*
YIELD: *approximately 1⅛ cup*

In a small saucepan over low heat or in a double boiler, warm the base oils and cocoa butter until the coconut oil and cocoa butter have just melted. Remove from heat and stir the mixture with a spoon or small whisk for 15 seconds to thoroughly blend. Add the fragrance oil (if desired) and stir again.

Pour the blend into a storage container and cap when almost cool. Allow the mixture to thicken for 12 hours before use.

Note: If the temperature of your storage area is above 76°F, the product will maintain a liquid consistency. If it's below 76°F, it will be firmer. To soften before use, set container in a shallow pan of hot water for 10 to 20 minutes. Shake bottle vigorously prior to each use.

No refrigeration is required, but for maximum freshness and potency, please use within 2 years.

APPLICATION TIPS: Apply this oil immediately after a bath or shower to seal in moisture and prevent evaporation before heading into the sun. It's very concentrated; begin with 1 teaspoon. Also remember to apply it during and after sun exposure.

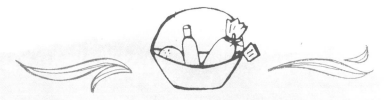

Sun Sense Gift Idea

Know any sun worshippers? Everyone does! Often by March 1 they're outside trying to get a jump on their summer tan — even if there's still snow on the ground! Many of these people aren't too keen on using sunscreen, either, but I'm sure they would appreciate a bottle of your freshly made, low-SPF Tropical Creamy Body Oil.

- Fill an 8-ounce plastic squeeze bottle with your wonderful-smelling creation.
- Apply a decorative, instructional label.
- Tie a piece of twine and a couple of seashells around the top.

Blue Chamomile and Olive Body Butter

This recipe in its original form offers anti-inflammatory care for environmentally damaged and sunburned skin, but to give it a low SPF (the original recipe has none) and enhance its sun-protection properties, substitute unrefined sesame base oil or a blend of 50 percent neem base oil and 50 percent jojoba base oil for the extra-virgin olive base oil.

See recipe under Body Moisturizers: Creams, Butters, and Balms, page 224.

APPLICATION TIPS: Apply before, during, and after sun exposure. It helps heal and condition skin overexposed to the elements.

Cocoa Butter Creamy Lotion for Face and Body

This ultra-thick lotion is a fantastic natural sun-care formula, but to give it a low SPF (the original recipe has none), substitute unrefined sesame base oil for the soybean, almond, apricot kernel, or macadamia nut base oil. Omit the essential oils except vanilla, if desired.

See recipe under Face Moisturizers, page 196.

APPLICATION TIPS: Apply before, during, and after sun exposure to insure soft, supple skin.

ALOE AFTER-SUN RELIEF SPRAY

This blend, with hydrating and anti-inflammatory properties, soothes and rejuvenates skin damaged by sunburn and windburn. It doubles as an anti-itch and
healing spray for those suffering from all manner of skin irritation and bug bites.

1 cup aloe vera juice
20 drops lavender essential oil
10 drops rosemary (chemotype
   verbenon) essential oil

RECOMMENDED FOR: *all skin types,
especially environmentally irritated and
abused skin*
USE: *as necessary*
PREP TIME: *approximately 5 minutes*
BLENDING TOOLS: *shake vigorously
before each use*
STORE IN: *plastic or dark glass spray or
spritzer bottle*
YIELD: *approximately 1 cup*

Place all ingredients in a storage container and shake well to blend.
Please keep refrigerated and use within 4 to 6 months.

APPLICATION TIPS: Spray on skin as often as necessary.

SUNBURN RELIEF SUGGESTIONS

- Add 2 cups apple cider vinegar to cool bath water and soak for
  10 to 20 minutes.
- Apply cold aloe vera gel or juice directly to sunburn as often as
  needed to ease pain and rehydrate damaged tissue.
- Apply cold, strong, regular black pekoe tea directly to sunburn
  with soaked cotton pads. Repeat as needed.
- Spray chilled lavender or chamomile hydrosol directly onto sunburned areas to help relieve inflammation.

Body Exfoliants: Be Smooth and Glow

The skin of a polished, routinely exfoliated body is not only more comfortable to live in than it's dry, scaly counterpart, but it also has a healthy radiance, retains more moisture and flexibility, and remains youthful-looking longer.

As we've learned, the epidermis, or outermost layer of your skin, sheds millions of dead cells daily. The rate at which your body renews its skin slows as you age, however, so exfoliation becomes increasingly important to maintaining healthy, supple skin. If these dead cells remain on your skin, they can form a thick layer of buildup, creating a semi-impenetrable barrier to applied moisturizers. Such thirsty skin is prone to wrinkles and rapidly shows its age. Manual exfoliation aids the body in its natural shedding process. It also helps loosen ingrown hairs, stimulate circulation, and lift away dirt and sebum without the use of drying soap.

You'll notice that some of the recipes that follow include salt and some call for sugar. Sea salt is healing to the skin when used in moderation, but it can sting and dehydrate irritated, sensitive, sunburned, windburned, thin, mature, or fair skin. Skin that has just been shaved or waxed will burn when salt is applied. I use a salt scrub when my skin is particularly dirty or I really need to slough rough knees, elbows, palms, and feet. It can be used all over if you are able to tolerate it without discomfort.

As my primary scrub base, however, I prefer granulated brown or white sugar, since it never stings — but it too can be physically irritating to sensitive and thin skin, unless used with great care. In addition to being an abrasive exfoliant, sugar acts on a chemical level: It contains natural glycolic acid, an ingredient that dissolves dead cells and clarifies skin.

Note: The following scrub recipes are for your body only and are not to be used on your delicate face, throat, or décolleté. (Scrub recipes for these areas can be found under Exfoliant Facial Scrubs on page 175.) Be careful not to abuse and irritate your skin by scrubbing too vigorously. A gentle touch is all that's needed.

Some have asked me if scrub ingredients can clog the shower drain. I've never had a problem with this, provided I routinely keep the drain clean and free of hair buildup. The salt and sugar dissolve in water within a minute or two of application and the spices, clay, ground oats, and ground sunflower seeds absorb water and become a slurry that simply rinses off and easily flows down the drain.

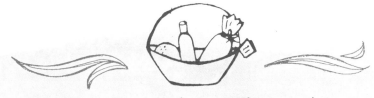

Body Exfoliant Gift Idea

Fragrant salt and sugar body scrubs will leave even the driest, scaly skin smooth and soft and luxuriously polished. Scrubs are a welcome gift to receive at the end of summer and during the winter, when skin can be its most "lizardy."

- Try to discover the recipient's favorite natural fragrance and scent the scrub accordingly.
- Package one of the following recipes in a wide-mouth, glass jar or in an attractive plastic jar.
- Tie a piece of twine or raffia with a decorative label and clearly detailed instructions to the top and your gift is ready to give.

Simply Sweet and Spicy Brown Sugar Body Polish

This scrub is a true sensory delight for the spice lover. The stimulating aroma subtly lingers long after the sugar has been rinsed away. A particularly inviting scrub for men, it provides effective exfoliation and deeply moisturized smoothness to skin yet is not femininely fragranced.

1	cup brown sugar
1	cup white granulated sugar
¾	cup almond, soybean, hazelnut, or macadamia nut base oil
2	teaspoons cinnamon, powdered
2	teaspoons ginger, powdered
2	teaspoons nutmeg, powdered
40	drops cardamom essential oil

RECOMMENDED FOR: *all skin types except acneic (use with care on sensitive and environmentally damaged skin)*
USE: *1 to 2 times per week*
FOLLOW WITH: *moisturizer if necessary*
PREP TIME: *approximately 10 minutes*
BLENDING TOOLS: *medium-sized bowl and whisk*
STORE IN: *wide mouthed plastic or glass jar*
YIELD: *slightly more than 2 cups*

In a medium-sized bowl, combine all ingredients except the essential oil. Using a whisk, blend ingredients thoroughly, making sure to break up any lumps of brown sugar or spice. Add the essential oil drop by drop, blending after each addition.

Spoon into a storage container with a tight-fitting lid.

No refrigeration is required, but for maximum freshness and fragrance, please use within 6 months.

APPLICATION TIPS: Massage approximately ¼ to ½ cup of scrub onto premoistened skin using circular motions. Rinse.

COCONUT AND VANILLA BROWN SUGAR
BODY BUFF

The aroma of this scrub is so richly tropical! It's a delightful skin polishing formula to use year-round, but especially when you wish you were in the balmy, breezy, warm tropics.

1¼ cups brown or raw sugar
6–8 tablespoons coconut base oil
   (extra-virgin; unrefined)
15–20 drops vanilla essential
   oil (or substitute vanilla
   fragrance or flavoring oil.
   Follow package directions
   for proper measurements.)

RECOMMENDED FOR: *all skin types except acneic (use with care on sensitive and environmentally damaged skin)*
USE: *1 to 2 times per week*
FOLLOW WITH: *moisturizer if necessary*
PREP TIME: *approximately 10 minutes*
BLENDING TOOLS: *medium-sized bowl and small whisk*
STORE IN: *wide mouthed plastic or glass jar*
YIELD: *approximately 1¼ cups*

In a medium-sized bowl, combine sugar and coconut base oil. If the temperature of your house is below 76°F and the coconut oil is solid, warm it over very low heat until it's just melted, then blend with the sugar using a small whisk, making sure to break up any lumps of sugar. Add the essential oil drop by drop, blending after each addition.

Spoon into a storage container with a tight-fitting lid.

Note: At temperatures below 76°F, this scrub will harden because of its coconut base oil content, but it can still be scooped out of the container with a spoon and applied to skin. Coconut oil will melt upon contact with body temperature.

No refrigeration is required, but for maximum freshness and fragrance, please use within 6 months.

APPLICATION TIPS: Massage approximately ¼ to ½ cup of scrub onto premoistened skin using circular motions. Rinse.

Basic Herbal Body Cleansing Exfoliant and Soap Substitute

I use this formula often when my skin is dry and I want to avoid soap. It thoroughly cleanses without stripping natural oils, leaving skin feeling fresh and soft. It doubles as a gentle, soap-free facial cleanser for all skin types and can be used as a mask.

½ cup ground oatmeal or oat flour

½ cup lavender buds, powdered, or ¼ cup dried, ground orange peel

½ cup sunflower seed meal

½ cup white clay

40 drops lavender or sweet orange essential oil (optional)

Purified water or milk

RECOMMENDED FOR: *all skin types*
USE: *daily if desired*
FOLLOW WITH: *moisturizer*
PREP TIME: *approximately 10 to 15 minutes (if meals are ground ahead of time)*
BLENDING TOOLS: *medium-sized bowl and whisk*
STORE IN: *wide mouthed plastic or glass jar or tin (dry ingredients and essential oil only)*
YIELD: *approximately 2 cups*

Place all dry ingredients in a medium-sized bowl. Using a whisk, gently stir to evenly blend. Add the essential oil drop by drop, gently whisking after each addition.

Spoon mix into a storage container.

No refrigeration is required, but for maximum freshness and fragrance, please use within 6 months.

To mix scrub for use, place ¼ to ½ cup of scrub into a small bowl and add enough water or milk to form a spreadable paste.

APPLICATION TIPS: Moisten skin so that it is damp. Massage scrub over entire body using circular motions for at least 2 minutes in order to soften dry skin cells. Rinse.

TO USE AS A FACIAL MASK: Simply apply a thin layer, allow it to dry for 20 minutes, then rinse with warm water and pat dry.

SALT OF THE EARTH BODY SCRUB

This is an ultra-invigorating blend, perfect to use in the morning as a wake-me-up, skin-sparkling scrub. It enlivens all the senses!

2   cups sea salt (preferably finely ground, but regular granular will do)
¾   cup extra-virgin olive base oil or base oil of choice
40–60 drops peppermint, spearmint, grapefruit, geranium, or rosemary (chemotype *verbenon*) essential oil

RECOMMENDED FOR: *all skin types except acneic (use with care on sensitive and environmentally damaged skin)*
USE: *1 to 2 times per week*
FOLLOW WITH: *moisturizer if necessary*
PREP TIME: *approximately 10 minutes*
BLENDING TOOLS: *medium-sized bowl and whisk*
STORE IN: *wide mouthed plastic or glass jar*
YIELD: *approximately 2 cups*

In a medium-sized bowl, combine the sea salt and the base oil. Using a whisk, stir to blend. Add the essential oil drop by drop, blending after each addition.

Spoon into a storage container with a tight-fitting lid.

No refrigeration is required, but for maximum freshness and fragrance, please use within 6 months.

APPLICATION TIPS: Massage approximately ¼ to ½ cup of scrub onto premoistened skin using circular motions. Rinse.

Aromatic and Deodorizing Body Powders

Talc is often the first ingredient that we associate with body powder. Though inexpensive, talc can be irritating to the lungs and frequently contains traces of arsenic. Most commercial body powders use 100 percent talc. Deodorizing body powders and baby powders often contain a blend of talc, baking soda, and cornstarch or can be pure cornstarch with a fragrance additive.

My favorite powder consists of two parts cornstarch, one part white clay, one part baking soda, and one-half part powdered rose petals, with lavender and neroli essential oils added for fragrance. Sometimes, for simplicity and speed, I just use 100 percent cornstarch as my base.

Other excellent base powder choices to use alone or in combination in place of talc include:

- arrowroot powder
- baking soda
- chickpea flour
- corn flour
- cornstarch
- French green clay, finely ground
- oat flour
- powdered calendula blossoms
- powdered chamomile flowers
- powdered lavender buds
- powdered neem herb
- powdered rose petals
- rice flour
- white clay, finely ground

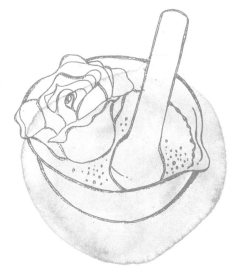

The following recipes are blends that I enjoy, but feel free to substitute or experiment with other base powder choices that are more to your liking.

Body Powder Gift Idea

Herbal body powders make great Christmas stocking stuffers and Mother's Day, wedding, or baby shower gifts.

- Make one of the following recipes and divide it into three or four portions.
- Find a decorative tin; a round, antique glass powder jar; or a small wooden or cardboard powder box that you've stenciled with a unique design and add enough (approximately ¾ to 1 cup) of the herbal powder recipe so that it fills two-thirds of the container.
- Place a satin-backed puff or small, fuzzy fluff brush inside and top the container with a bow and personalized label.
- Some craft stores carry shaker containers, which are always nice for storing body powder, too. If you don't want to package your gift in one of these, you could include one for use.

Lavender Powder

This recipe makes a light, lovely, old-fashioned, floral-scented body powder. It's especially wonderful to use on baby girls; it leaves behind a sweet, delicate, feminine aroma.

1   cup arrowroot
1   cup cornstarch
1   cup white clay
½   cup lavender buds, finely powdered
½   cup rose petals, finely powdered
200 drops of lavender or geranium essential oil

RECOMMENDED FOR: *all skin types*
USE: *as desired*
PREP TIME: *approximately 20 minutes, plus 3 days for fragrance to synergize*
BLENDING TOOLS: *large bowl and whisk or food processor, mortar and pestle*
STORE IN: *zip-seal plastic bag, wooden or cardboard box, tin, plastic or glass jar, or shaker container*
YIELD: *approximately 4 cups*

Combine all ingredients except the essential oil in a large bowl or food processor. Stir slowly with a whisk or whirl in the food processor for 15 seconds until well blended. Using a mortar and pestle, combine the essential oil drop by drop with 6 or 7 tablespoons of the powder mix until the oil is absorbed. Add this oil mixture to the remaining powder and whisk the mixture slowly (to avoid making too much dust) or shake vigorously in a large container with a tight-fitting lid. If using a food processor, whirl for 15 seconds to blend.

Store the powder in an airtight storage container in a cool, dark place for 3 days to allow the scent of the essential oil and the flowers to permeate the mixture. Package the powder in smaller containers if desired.

No refrigeration is required, but for maximum fragrance and freshness, please use within 1 year.

APPLICATION TIPS: Apply as you would any body powder — by sprinkling or "puffing" over entire body or only certain areas.

Vanilla Spice Powder

*T*his mixture has a round, full, sensual, spicy fragrance. It's quite heavenly. If you omit the vanilla beans and vanilla essential oil, many men will find this powder to their liking. Caution: *Powder may stain light-colored clothing.*

1½ cups cornstarch

1 cup rice flour

½ cup white clay

3 vanilla beans, chopped into ¼-inch pieces

1 tablespoon cinnamon powder

1 tablespoon nutmeg powder

50 drops **each** of the following essential oils: vanilla; cinnamon bark (substitute sweet orange if skin is sensitive); cardamom

RECOMMENDED FOR: *all skin types*
USE: *as desired*
PREP TIME: *approximately 20 to 30 minutes, plus 3 days for fragrance to synergize*
BLENDING TOOLS: *large bowl and whisk or food processor, mortar and pestle*
STORE IN: *zip-seal plastic bag, wooden or cardboard box, tin, plastic or glass jar, or shaker container*
YIELD: *approximately 3⅛ cups*

Combine all ingredients except the essential oils in a large bowl or food processor. Stir slowly with a whisk or whirl in the food processor for 15 seconds until well blended. The vanilla beans will remain in pieces. Using a mortar and pestle, combine the essential oils drop by drop with 6 or 7 tablespoons of powder until the oil is absorbed. Add this oil mixture to the remaining powder and whisk the mixture slowly or shake vigorously in a large container with a tight-fitting lid. If using a food processor, whirl for 15 seconds to blend.

Store powder in an airtight storage container in a cool, dark place for 3 days to allow the scent of the essential oils, spices, and vanilla beans to permeate the mixture. Package the powder in smaller containers if desired.

No refrigeration is required, but please use within 1 year.

APPLICATION TIPS: Apply as you would any body powder — by sprinkling or "puffing" over entire body or only certain areas.

BABY POWDER

This very gentle powder has only a hint of fragrance. It's perfect for keeping baby's (and adult's) sensitive skin soft and dry.

1½ cups arrowroot

½ cup baking soda

½ cup calendula, chamomile, or elder flowers, very finely powdered

½ cup rice flour or cornstarch

20 drops Roman chamomile, lavender, or sweet orange essential oil

RECOMMENDED FOR: *all skin types*
USE: *as desired*
PREP TIME: *approximately 15 minutes, plus 3 days for fragrance to synergize*
BLENDING TOOLS: *large bowl and whisk or food processor, mortar and pestle*
STORE IN: *zip-seal plastic bag, wooden or cardboard box, tin, plastic or glass jar, or shaker container*
YIELD: *approximately 3 cups*

Combine all ingredients except the essential oil in a large bowl or food processor. Stir slowly with a whisk or whirl in the food processor for 15 seconds until well blended. Using a mortar and pestle, combine the essential oil drop by drop with 6 or 7 tablespoons of powder until the oil is absorbed. Add this oil mixture to the remaining powder and whisk the mixture slowly (to avoid making too much dust) or shake vigorously in a large container with a tight-fitting lid. If using a food processor, whirl for 15 seconds to blend.

Store powder in an airtight storage container in a cool, dark place for 3 days to allow the scent of the essential oil and flowers to permeate the mixture. Package the powder in smaller containers if desired.

No refrigeration is required, but for maximum fragrance and freshness, please use within 1 year.

APPLICATION TIPS: Apply as you would any body powder — by sprinkling or "puffing" over the entire body or only certain areas.

REFRESHING BODY AND FOOT POWDER

This is a refreshing, stimulating, absorbent powder to use before and after exercise, especially in hot weather. It's a perfect choice for deodorizing tired, smelly feet and keeping underarms dry.

1 cup baking soda
1 cup white clay
1½ cups arrowroot
¼ cup orange peel, very finely powdered
¼ cup peppermint, very finely powdered
100 drops peppermint essential oil
100 drops lemon essential oil

RECOMMENDED FOR: *all skin types*
USE: *as desired*
PREP TIME: *approximately 20 minutes, plus 3 days for fragrance to synergize*
BLENDING TOOLS: *large bowl and whisk or food processor, mortar and pestle*
STORE IN: *zip-seal plastic bag, wooden or cardboard box, tin, plastic or glass jar, or shaker container*
YIELD: *approximately 4 cups*

Combine all ingredients except the essential oils in a large bowl or food processor. Stir slowly with a whisk or whirl in the food processor for 15 seconds until well blended. Using a mortar and pestle, combine the essential oils drop by drop with 2 or 3 tablespoons of powder until the oil is absorbed. Add this oil mixture to the remaining powder and whisk the mixture slowly (to avoid making too much dust) or shake vigorously in a large container with a tight-fitting lid. If using a food processor, whirl for 15 seconds to blend.

Store powder in an airtight storage container in a cool, dark place for 3 days to allow the scent of the essential oils and herbs to permeate the mixture. Package the powder in smaller containers if desired.

No refrigeration is required, but for maximum fragrance and freshness, please use within 1 year.

APPLICATION TIPS: Apply as you would any body powder — by sprinkling or "puffing" over the entire body or only certain areas.

Rosemary and Thyme Body Powder

*T*his powder, enjoyed by both men and women, has an herbal, green aroma with antiseptic and antibacterial properties. It's quite effective as a natural underarm deodorant when commercial deodorants must be avoided.

1¾ cup cornstarch

¾ cup baking soda

¼ cup thyme, very finely powdered

¼ cup white clay

100 drops rosemary (chemotype *verbenon*) essential oil

50 drops thyme (chemotype *linalol*) essential oil

RECOMMENDED FOR: *all skin types, especially those sensitive to chemical-based deodorants*
USE: *as desired*
PREP TIME: *approximately 20 minutes, plus 3 days for fragrance to synergize*
BLENDING TOOLS: *large bowl and whisk or food processor, mortar and pestle*
STORE IN: *zip-seal plastic bag, wooden or cardboard box, tin, plastic or glass jar, or shaker container*
YIELD: *approximately 3 cups*

Combine all ingredients except the essential oils in a large bowl or food processor. Stir slowly with a whisk or whirl in the food processor for 15 seconds until well blended. Using a mortar and pestle, combine the essential oils drop by drop with 6 or 7 tablespoons of powder until the oil is absorbed. Add this oil mixture to the remaining powder and whisk the mixture slowly (to avoid making too much dust) or shake vigorously in a large container with a tight-fitting lid. If using a food processor, whirl for 15 seconds to blend.

Store powder in an airtight storage container in a cool, dark place for 3 days to allow the scent of the essential oils and thyme to permeate the mixture. Package the powder in smaller containers if desired.

No refrigeration is required, but please use within 1 year.

APPLICATION TIPS: Apply as you would any body powder — by sprinkling or "puffing" over the entire body or only certain areas.

FRESH AND DRY ALL-DAY POWDER

*T*his powder is especially effective as a feminine hygiene product and can be safely used in women's more delicate and sweat-prone areas. If you want a more cooling, medicinal powder, use tea tree essential oil instead of sweet orange oil.

¼ cup white clay

¾ cup plus 2 tablespoons baking soda

¾ cup cornstarch

2 tablespoons myrrh, powdered

50 drops sweet orange essential oil (or tea tree essential oil for a more medicinal, deodorizing, antifungal formula)

RECOMMENDED FOR: *all skin types*
USE: *as desired*
PREP TIME: *approximately 15 minutes, plus 3 days for fragrance to synergize*
BLENDING TOOLS: *medium-sized bowl and whisk or food processor, mortar and pestle*
STORE IN: *zip-seal plastic bag, wooden or cardboard box, tin, plastic or glass jar, or shaker container*
YIELD: *approximately 2 cups*

Combine all ingredients except the essential oil in a medium-sized bowl or food processor. Stir slowly with a whisk or whirl in the food processor for 15 seconds until well blended. Using a mortar and pestle, combine the essential oil drop by drop with 3 or 4 tablespoons of powder until the oil is absorbed. Add this oil mixture to the remaining powder and whisk the mixture slowly or shake vigorously in a container with a tight-fitting lid. If using a food processor, whirl for 15 seconds to blend.

Store powder in an airtight storage container in a cool, dark place for 3 days to allow the scent of the essential oils and myrrh to permeate the mixture. Package the powder in smaller containers if desired.

No refrigeration is required, but please use within 1 year.

APPLICATION TIPS: Apply as you would any body powder — by sprinkling or "puffing" over the entire body or only certain areas.

Foot Care: Feelin' Foot Loose and Fancy Free

Your feet were designed to be strong, support your weight, and provide leverage while you walk. Though some think feet are a beautiful part of the body, most of us would rather hide our tootsies than show them off!

As an esthetician, I have heard many complaints from clients regarding their feet: "They constantly hurt," "My calluses are so thick I have to cut them with a knife," "My toenails are getting narrow, thick, and ugly," "I'm constantly battling foot odor and sweaty feet." Most of these problems are easily rectified.

One important question can begin to address these concerns: What kind of shoes do you most often wear? Many women's shoes are designed purely for fashion, not comfort. Ill-fitting footwear can cause myriad foot problems. You may find that purchasing properly fitting, attractive, "sensible" shoes will solve problems of corns, calluses, chronic aches, and tiredness. More than ever before, today there are many shoe styles created with both your comfort and fashion in mind.

Foot odor, a common and embarrassing problem, can usually be remedied by wearing natural fiber or moisture-wicking socks and shoes that breathe. If you have other foot problems, such as bunions, hammertoe, fallen arches, excessive perspiration and odor, or toenail fungus that won't go away, see a podiatrist, a physician specializing in foot disorders.

For basic care and preventive maintenance, treat your feet with the following recipes designed to bring relief to your tired, rough, itchy, dry, thickened, abused, neglected, and odoriferous dogs. Many of the recipes require the use of a foot tub, found at your local grocery or hardware store. It's essentially a plastic dishpan approximately 5 inches deep, 12 inches wide, and 12 to 23 inches long. If you really want to pamper your feet, consider a foot tub with mini-jacuzzi action and vibrating foot pads, available from most department stores and better drug stores.

FOOT-CARE TIPS: *Foot rollers* are available in health food stores, online, and in shops that sell bath products. They are wonderful for relieving sore, tired feet. I prefer the wooden ones that have raised ridges from one end to the other. And remember: A foot massage is a luxury to receive! Massage your loved one's clean feet with any base oil (neem, though strongly scented, is particularly good for feet suffering from fissures, calluses, or hard-to-heal toenail disorders) mixed with a few drops of your favorite essential oil. This is a great way to spend the evening with your "sole" mate!

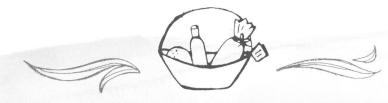

Foot Care Gift Idea

- Double or triple the Foot Scrub recipe (page 272; dry ingredients and essential oil only).
- Package it in a decorative tin, jar, or zip-seal bag placed inside a cardboard or wooden box. For an artistic touch, stencil some footprints on the tin or box.
- Whatever packaging you choose, be sure to label the container and include directions for use.
- A nice accompaniment is a ¼-ounce bottle of lemon or peppermint essential oil inside the container or attached to the outside with a ribbon.

Foot Scrub

This scrub is quick and easy to make and leaves feet feeling soft, smooth, tingly, and refreshed.

¼ cup cornmeal
¼ cup ground oatmeal
1 tablespoon sea or table salt
Purified or tap water
A few drops lemon or
  peppermint essential oil

RECOMMENDED FOR: *rough, dry, callused feet*
USE: *daily or as needed*
FOLLOW WITH: *moisturizer*
PREP TIME: *approximately 5 minutes (if oatmeal is ground ahead of time)*
BLENDING TOOLS: *spoon and small bowl*
STORE IN: *do not store; mix as needed*
YIELD: *1 treatment*

Combine dry ingredients in a small bowl with enough water to form a creamy, gritty paste. Add a few drops of the essential oil and stir again.

APPLICATION TIPS: Sit on the edge of the bathtub or on a bench in the shower and massage your feet with this mixture — really scrub all those rough areas and between toes. I find this quite invigorating. Rinse and dry thoroughly and follow with an application of a thick moisturizing cream combined with a few drops of either essential oil.

Note: Make sure to clean the bathtub right after this procedure; the cornmeal might swell and clog the drain.

FOOT SOOTHER

This recipe softens leathery feet, deodorizes, and helps to relieve the itchiness of athlete's foot. Following this foot soak, use a pumice stone or pediwand to buff away any softened calluses.

Foot tub

2 cups apple cider vinegar, raw or processed

2 tablespoons vegetable glycerin

RECOMMENDED FOR: *dry, rough, odorous, or itchy feet*
USE: *daily or as desired*
FOLLOW WITH: *moisturizer and foot powder if desired*
PREP TIME: *approximately 5 minutes*
BLENDING TOOLS: *swish feet in tub to mix ingredients*
STORE IN: *do not store; mix as needed*
YIELD: *1 treatment*

Place ingredients into the foot tub with enough water, warm or cold, to cover your feet and ankles. Swish with feet to blend.

APPLICATION TIPS: Soak feet for 15 to 20 minutes. Pat dry and follow with a coating of moisturizer.

FOOT REFRESHER

The foot exercise and muscle stimulation combined with one of these invigorating essential oils and Epsom salt refresh and relieve achy, swollen feet. This soak is recommended for athletes or those who are on their feet all day.

Foot tub

½ cup Epsom salt

5–10 drops of lemon, tangerine, peppermint, spearmint, rosemary (chemotype *verbenon*), juniper, or eucalyptus radiata essential oil

2–3 cups medium-sized marbles

RECOMMENDED FOR: *tired, achy, swollen feet*
USE: *daily or as desired*
FOLLOW WITH: *moisturizer and foot powder if desired*
PREP TIME: *approximately 10 minutes*
BLENDING TOOLS: *swish feet in tub to mix ingredients*
STORE IN: *do not store; mix as needed*
YIELD: *1 treatment*

Place the Epsom salt and the essential oil of choice into the foot tub with enough comfortably hot or cold-as-you-can-stand water to cover your feet and ankles. Swish with feet to blend. Next, add enough marbles to almost cover the bottom of the tub.

APPLICATION TIPS: Soak feet for 15 to 20 minutes while gently rolling them back and forth over the marbles. Occasionally, grasp and release marbles with toes. This action stretches and relaxes the feet. Roughly rub feet dry and apply a soothing lotion mixed with a few drops of one of the chosen essential oils.

FOOT DEODORIZER

These specific herbs and essential oils all have astringent, pore-tightening properties and are known deodorizers that truly freshen sweaty or odorous feet.

Foot tub

6 quarts water (tap water is fine)

½ cup sage, peppermint,
   or rosemary leaves

½ cup baking soda

5–10 drops rosemary (chemotype
   verbenon), sweet orange,
   peppermint, tea tree, or
   eucalyptus radiata essential oil

RECOMMENDED FOR: *foot odor,
sweaty feet*
USE: *daily or as needed*
FOLLOW WITH: *moisturizer and foot
powder if desired*
PREP TIME: *approximately 40 minutes*
BLENDING TOOLS: *swish feet in tub to
mix ingredients*
STORE IN: *do not store; mix as needed*
YIELD: *1 treatment*

In a large pot, bring the water to a boil, remove
from heat, and add the herb of choice. Cover and
steep for 30 minutes. Strain into the foot tub.
Add baking soda and the essential oil and swish
with feet to blend.

APPLICATION TIPS: Soak feet for approximately 15 to 20 minutes. Towel dry and follow
with a coating of moisturizer.

SIMPLY SOFT SOLES

A generous application of
pure coconut oil or shea butter to your feet on a daily
basis will go a long way
toward ensuring that they
are protected from skin
damaging dryness and its
resultant roughness, fissures,
and general discomfort. This
is a wonderfully inexpensive
and highly effective way to
treat your feet!

Feelin' Fresh Foot Powder

This recipe makes a very effective deodorizing foot and underarm powder. It can also be used to prevent diaper rash on baby bottoms — but omit the essential oil, please.

1   cup baking soda
1   cup cornstarch
2   tablespoons white clay
2   tablespoons zinc oxide powder
100 drops lemongrass, thyme (chemotype *linalol*), sweet orange, tangerine, peppermint, or tea tree essential oil

RECOMMENDED FOR: *prevention of foot odor and dampness*
USE: *daily or as needed*
PREP TIME: *approximately 15 minutes, plus 3 days for fragrance to synergize*
BLENDING TOOLS: *medium-sized bowl and whisk or food processor*
STORE IN: *plastic or glass jar or shaker container*
YIELD: *approximately 2¼ cups*

In a medium-sized bowl, gently mix dry ingredients using a whisk or place in the food processor and pulse a few times. Add the essential oil a few drops at a time and blend with the whisk, or continue pulsing the food processor as you add the drops.

Store powder in an airtight storage container in a cool, dark place for 3 days to allow the essential oil fragrance and deodorizing properties to permeate the mixture. After this time, package the blend in small shaker containers or reuse clean spice shaker jars for ease of application.

No refrigeration is required, but for maximum fragrance and potency, please use within 1 year.

APPLICATION TIPS: Sprinkle into shoes and socks once or twice daily or simply sprinkle onto dry, bare feet whenever desired.

Fungus Treatment Oil Drops

K eep in mind that fungus is often difficult to eradicate, even with prescription drugs, so months of consistent treatment — whether with a natural remedy, over-the-counter medication, or prescription — is warranted.

20 drops tea tree essential oil
15 drops thyme (chemotype linalol) essential oil
10 drops German chamomile essential oil
5   drops clove essential oil
1   tablespoon hazelnut base oil
1   tablespoon neem base oil

RECOMMENDED FOR: *athlete's foot, toenail fungus, itchy feet*
USE: *twice per day*
PREP TIME: *approximately 15 minutes, plus 24 hours to synergize*
BLENDING TOOLS: *shake storage bottle before each use*
STORE IN: *dark glass bottle with glass dropper top*
YIELD: *2 tablespoons or 1 ounce*

Add the essential oils, drop by drop, directly into a storage bottle. Next, add the base oils. Screw on the bottle's dropper top, wrap your hand around the bottle, and shake the bottle vigorously for 2 minutes to blend all ingredients and warm to body temperature.

Place the bottle in a dark location that's between 60 and 80°F for 24 hours to allow the oils to synergize.

No refrigeration is necessary, but for maximum fragrance and potency, please use within 6 months.

APPLICATION TIPS: For athlete's foot or any other fungal affliction that affects the entire foot, place 10–20 drops into your palm and massage thoroughly into the foot. Concentrate on the area between the toes and around the cuticles. If only one foot is affected, treat the other one anyway — fungus can spread. If you're suffering from toenail fungus, place 1 drop onto each toenail and massage in. Perform treatments twice per day on clean feet until the fungus disappears.

Callus Remover

*I*f this recipe and procedure are used on a consistent basis, your feet will become softer and healthier and unsightly calluses will be a problem of the past. You might just decide you want to show off those tootsies!

Foot tub
½ cup baking soda
½ cup sea or table salt
Pumice stone (synthetic or real) or pediwand

RECOMMENDED FOR: *rough, callused feet*
USE: *daily or as needed*
FOLLOW WITH: *moisturizer or favorite balm*
PREP TIME: *approximately 5 minutes*
BLENDING TOOLS: *swish feet in tub to mix ingredients*
STORE IN: *do not store; mix as needed*
YIELD: *1 treatment*

Fill the foot tub with comfortably warm or hot water to cover your feet and ankles, add the baking soda and salt, and swish with feet to dissolve ingredients.

APPLICATION TIPS: Soak feet for 15 or 20 minutes or longer if calluses are very thick. Remove one foot from the water and, while still wet, gently scrub calluses with the exfoliating tool of choice. When the loose skin begins building up on the scrubbing tool, dip it and your foot back into the foot tub, rinse, and begin again if necessary. Repeat the process with other foot. Roughly rub feet dry and apply a thick cream, your favorite balm, or nonpetroleum jelly, then don natural-fiber socks. This final application will continue to soften your feet throughout the day or overnight. You can also follow this procedure while taking a bath, after your feet have become soft.

Beautifying Hand and Nail Treatments

Next time you're at a social function, take a look at the hands around you. Can you tell what kind of work they do just by looking at their hands? A mechanic's hands and nails will frequently be grease-stained. An accountant, attorney, or administrative assistant's will be smooth and soft, typically with well-groomed nails. A full-time mother with several children and a small garden will probably have hands sporting short nails and dry skin and cuticles. A carpenter, mason, or farmer may have rough, cracked, suntanned hands with hard fingernails and thick calluses.

We tend to pay so much attention to our face and hair but often neglect one of our most expressive features: our hands. They are constantly exposed to the elements: sun, wind, heat, cold, harsh cleansers, dirt, grease, and so on, and are one of the first places on our body to show age.

You can fight the ravages of time and the elements on your hands by remembering to take a few important steps each day: Apply moisturizer *frequently,* wear rubber gloves when hands will be exposed to water or cleansers, and wear garden gloves when working outdoors. Don't forget to apply to your hands a natural sunscreen lotion with an SPF of 15 whenever you're in the sun. Sun damage can result in premature aging of the skin, blotchiness, dryness, and those dreaded dark brown liver spots.

The following recipes will help to soften and protect your hands and nails.

Hand and Nail Butter

This formula is rich, moisturizing, and healing for irritated, dry hands and nails, chapped lips, rough knees, elbows, and feet. It's particularly effective for the prevention of scar tissue formation (if formulated with carrot seed or rosemary essential oil) when consistently applied to fresh cuts and scrapes.

4 tablespoons almond base oil

2 tablespoons cocoa butter

1 tablespoon anhydrous lanolin

1 tablespoon beeswax (use 1½ tablespoons if you want a firmer consistency)

50 drops peppermint, carrot seed, rosemary (chemotype verbenon), geranium, lemon, or grapefruit essential oil (or any combination)

RECOMMENDED FOR: *everyone, especially those with dry, rough, chapped hands and cuticles*
USE: *daily or as desired*
PREP TIME: *approximately 30 minutes, plus 12 hours to completely set*
BLENDING TOOLS: *small whisk or spoon*
STORE IN: *plastic or glass jar or tin*
YIELD: *approximately ½ cup*

In a small saucepan over low heat or in a double boiler, warm all ingredients except the essential oil until the wax and cocoa butter are just melted. Remove from heat and stir a few times to blend. Add the essential oil, stir, and pour into storage container(s).

Lightly cover each container with a paper towel and allow the mixture to cool before capping. Cocoa butter takes a while to set up, so leave the product at room temperature for 12 hours before use. The finished formula will have a paste wax consistency.

Note: This formula may harden in cold weather but will soften upon contact with warm skin.

No refrigeration is required, but for maximum freshness and potency, please use within 1 year.

APPLICATION TIPS: Use this on hands and feet as an overnight softening treatment. Wear gloves or socks to seal in moisture and protect sheets.

FOR A NAIL AND CUTICLE TREATMENT: Soak clean fingertips in a bowl of warm water for 2 minutes to soften nail and cuticles. Pat dry. Apply a tiny dab of this butter onto the base of each nail and massage in. Using a small piece of cotton flannel, gently push back cuticles, and then lightly buff nails with the cloth. This treatment leaves fingertips soft and smooth.

For shiny nails, apply the butter as for the nail and cuticle treatment, but use a nail buffer instead of the cloth to polish nails gently to a soft sheen.

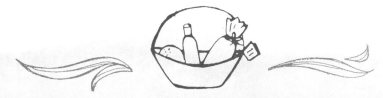

Hand and Nail Care Gift Idea

A small basket of hand and nail care products makes the perfect gift for those who work with their hands or frequently expose them to the elements.

- Fill a basket with a jar of Hand and Nail Butter (see recipe left), a 10- by 10-inch piece of pretty, soft cotton flannel (hem the edges first), a crystal nail file, clippers, and a nail buffer.
- Add or subtract any items to personalize the gift.
- A pair of white cotton gloves for an overnight treatment and a tube of natural sunscreen make a nice accompaniment.
- Include the recipe and application tips for the Hand and Nail Butter on a decorative tag, label, or card.

NOURISH-YOUR-NAILS OIL

This is a highly penetrable blend that moisturizes nails to maintain their strength and flexibility and prevent brittleness, dry peeling, and cracking.

20 drops lavender
essential oil

10 drops lemon
essential oil

1 tablespoon almond
base oil (or neem base oil
if you have nail fungus)

1 tablespoon jojoba
base oil

RECOMMENDED FOR: *everyone, especially those whose hands and nails are particularly dry or whose hands suffer from constant exposure to damaging elements (water, wind, sun, dirt, chemicals, soap, and so on.)*
USE: *nightly*
FOLLOW WITH: *hand cream or favorite balm if desired*
PREP TIME: *approximately 15 minutes, plus 24 hours to synergize*
BLENDING TOOLS: *shake storage bottle before each use*
STORE IN: *dark glass bottle with glass dropper top*
YIELD: *approximately 2 tablespoons*

Add the essential oils, drop by drop, directly into a storage bottle. Next, add the base oils. Screw on the bottle's dropper top, wrap your hand around the bottle, and shake the formula vigorously for 2 minutes to completely blend all ingredients and gently warm to body temperature.

Place the bottle in a dark location that's between 60 and 80°F for 24 hours so that the oils can synergize.

No refrigeration is required, but for maximum freshness and potency, please use within 6 months.

APPLICATION TIPS: Nightly, apply 1 drop to each nail and massage in with a soft flannel cloth (or your fingers) for approximately 1 minute per nail.

Castor Oil Soak

Thick, conditioning castor oil leaves behind a hard, shiny, protective residue on nails, helping to prevent environmental damage. It also strengthens nails and relieves drying and cracking of cuticles.

3–4 tablespoons castor base oil

10 drops frankincense essential oil (CO2 extract)

RECOMMENDED FOR: *dry, brittle, weak nails and cuticles*
USE: *daily or as desired*
FOLLOW WITH: *moisturizer or favorite balm*
PREP TIME: *approximately 5 minutes*
BLENDING TOOLS: *small bowl and spoon*
STORE IN: *small glass bowl with cover*
YIELD: *3 or 4 tablespoons or treatments*

In a small glass bowl, place all ingredients and mix them with a spoon. Cover the bowl tightly.

Refrigerate for up to 1 month, then discard.

APPLICATION TIPS: Set bowl of oil in a shallow hot-water bath for a few minutes until it is comfortably warm. Soak clean fingertips in oil for 5 to 10 minutes to soften nails and cuticles slightly. Pat dry. Using a small piece of cotton flannel, gently push back cuticles, and then lightly buff nails with the cloth. The same blend can be used for 3–4 treatments. Each treatment uses approximately 1 tablespoon of oil blend.

Skin Lightening Hand Pack

*I*f this recipe is used consistently twice per week, hand skin coloration and texture should take on a more uniform appearance. You'll see gradual fading of age spots and hyperpigmentation and should experience enhanced softness and smoothness. This formula doubles as a pore-refining, skin-lightening facial mask for all skin types except very sensitive skin. Simply follow the same directions as applying it to hands, but make sure to relax and recline while it dries on your face.

1 tablespoon fresh lemon juice *or* fresh, raw apple, pineapple, or strawberry pulp

2 tablespoons ground oatmeal

1 tablespoon plain yogurt

RECOMMENDED FOR: *sun-damaged, dry, unevenly colored hands*
USE: *2 times per week*
FOLLOW WITH: *moisturizer or sunscreen*
PREP TIME: *approximately 10 minutes*
BLENDING TOOLS: *mortar and pestle, small bowl and spoon*
STORE IN: *do not store; mix as needed*
YIELD: *1 treatment*

Squeeze the lemon to extract juice or use a mortar and pestle to mash until pulpy a small amount of chosen fresh fruit. There is no need to strain juice from pulp. In a small bowl, combine all ingredients to form a spreadable paste and allow it to thicken for 1 minute. If the paste is too thick, add a bit of water to thin it slightly; if it's too thin, add more ground oatmeal.

APPLICATION TIPS: Apply mixture to the backs of clean hands and allow it to dry for 20 to 30 minutes. Rinse with cool water. Pat almost dry and apply a good moisturizer, balm, or sunscreen.

HAND AND NAIL INFECTION-FIGHTING OIL

I like to keep a bottle of this spicy, infused oil next to the kitchen sink so that I can use it as a quick first-aid oil to doctor my hands whenever I cut myself and want to aid in the prevention of possible infection. The cloves add an analgesic and mildly antiseptic property. This oil also eliminates kitchen hand odors such as garlic and onion.

¼ cup almond, soybean, macadamia, hazelnut, jojoba, or apricot kernel base oil

40 whole cloves

RECOMMENDED FOR: *extremely dry, fissured, rough hands, knuckles, and cuticles or for minor scrapes and scratches*
USE: *daily or as needed*
FOLLOW WITH: *moisturizer if desired*
PREP TIME: *approximately 5 minutes, plus 1 month for cloves to infuse oil*
BLENDING TOOLS: *shake container before use*
STORE IN: *glass bottle with glass dropper top or small glass jar*
YIELD: *¼ cup or 2 ounces*

In a small jar with a tight-fitting lid (a baby food jar is perfect), mix the oil and the cloves.

Tighten the lid of the jar and place it in a warm sunny window for one month to allow the cloves to impart their healing properties to the oil. Remember to shake mixture daily. The oil will take on a slight amber color, depending on the type of base oil you chose.

At the end of the extraction period, strain the cloves and pour into a storage container.

No refrigeration is required, but for maximum freshness and potency, please use within 6 months.

APPLICATION TIPS: Simply apply a drop or two of the oil to minor skin injuries of the hands and nails or massage a small amount into damp hands as a moisturizing, healing treatment.

Baking Soda Hand Exfoliant

This exfoliant removes dead skin buildup, leaving hands soft, smooth, and ready to accept moisturizer. This recipe is effective yet extremely gentle and doubles as an exfoliant for the entire body (including the face) if made in a larger batch.

1 tablespoon baking soda

1 teaspoon favorite base oil

2 drops geranium, lavender, or sweet orange essential oil (optional)

RECOMMENDED FOR: *all hands, especially those that are dry, rough, dirty, and weather-beaten*
USE: *daily or as desired*
FOLLOW WITH: *moisturizer or favorite balm*
PREP TIME: *approximately 5 minutes*
BLENDING TOOLS: *small bowl and spoon*
STORE IN: *do not store; mix as needed*
YIELD: *1 treatment*

In a small bowl, stir together all ingredients until a spreadable, thick paste forms.

APPLICATION TIPS: Apply the paste to dry hands, covering all surfaces thoroughly. For about 2 minutes, briskly rub together your hands, making sure to massage paste between fingers, around nails and cuticles, and over the backs of hands. Rinse with warm water and apply favorite moisturizer or balm.

Herbal Oral Hygiene

Most commercial toothpastes contain abrasives, artificial sweeteners, sugar, foaming agents, detergents, and synthetic whitening agents or bleaches, many of which, over the years, can wear down tooth enamel, erode gum tissue, and be absorbed into your body through the lining of your mouth. Most mouthwashes are colored with artificial dyes, infused with bad-breath-masking, synthetic flavors, and contain irritating chemicals and preservatives.

It's easy to make effective, inexpensive, tasty, nontoxic alternatives to standard oral care products. Though they won't taste as sweet as their commercial cousins, the flavors will grow on you, and you may notice that your mouth feels cleaner and fresher longer without the use of chemicals. Try a gentle, natural approach to maintain strong teeth and healthy gums with these recipes.

Note: If you have chronic bad breath or dental problems, see a dental professional.

Oral Hygiene Gift Idea

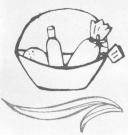

To give a lovely basket of dental hygiene products alone is akin to saying "Your breath smells horrible." Such a "gift" isn't advisable unless you want to embarrass the recipient! It's much better to give a sampler basket: a combination of body powder, massage oil, sleep balm, and an herbal mouthwash — to allow sampling your products without offense.

SODA AND SALT TOOTHPASTE

This is a simple, inexpensive, odor-eliminating, tooth-whitening, and highly effective formula. It leaves your mouth feeling super-clean. Note: *Cinnamon and clove essential oils may irritate sensitive gums and tongue.*

½ teaspoon baking soda
½ teaspoon sea salt, finely ground
1 drop peppermint, spearmint, sweet orange, clove, or cinnamon bark essential oil

A few drops tap water

RECOMMENDED FOR: *everyone*
USE: *daily*
FOLLOW WITH: *water rinse or mouthwash*
PREP TIME: *approximately 2 minutes*
BLENDING TOOLS: *small bowl, toothbrush, or small spoon*
STORE IN: *do not store; mix as needed*
YIELD: *1 treatment*

Combine ingredients in a small bowl and mix them thoroughly with a toothbrush, your finger, or a small spoon until a smooth, thick paste forms. The paste shouldn't be too runny; it has to stay on your toothbrush.

APPLICATION TIPS: Dip your toothbrush into the paste and use as you would regular commercial toothpaste.

Strawberry Tooth Brightener

Strawberries have a slight bleaching action and, if used daily, help to rid the teeth of tea, coffee, and cigarette stains. This treatment leaves your mouth feeling clean and tasting wonderful. A strawberry is much safer to use than lemon juice, which is much more acidic. When the fruit is in season, eating a bowl of strawberries daily is also another good way to brighten teeth and improve health.

1 medium-sized ripe strawberry

RECOMMENDED FOR: *everyone, especially those with stained teeth*
USE: *daily*
FOLLOW WITH: *water rinse or mouthwash*
PREP TIME: *approximately 2 minutes*
BLENDING TOOLS: *small bowl and fork or mortar and pestle, toothbrush*
STORE IN: *do not store; mix as needed*
YIELD: *1 treatment*

Remove the green top and stem first. Using a small bowl and fork or a mortar and pestle, mash the strawberry into a pulp.

APPLICATION TIPS: Dip your toothbrush into the pulp and brush normally. Rinse thoroughly.

TOOTH TWIG

This is definitely an old-fashioned way of brushing your teeth, but it's surprisingly effective. As a young girl, I learned about this old-time tooth-cleansing method from my grandfather, who told me much about Appalachian folk medicine during our many walks through his north Georgia farm and surrounding woodlands. It's great to use when you're wilderness camping and you've forgotten your regular toothbrush. This recyclable toothbrush is about as natural as they come!

4-inch–5-inch stiff twig from a sweet gum, sassafras, black gum (tupelo), or flowering dogwood tree (must be freshly cut)

RECOMMENDED FOR: *everyone*
USE: *daily*
FOLLOW WITH: *water rinse or mouthwash*
PREP TIME: *approximately 5 minutes*
STORE IN: *do not store or reuse*
YIELD: *1 treatment*

Peel the twig and chew on the end until it is frayed and soft. All of these tree varieties should taste slightly sweet.

APPLICATION TIPS: Dip the twig in a bit of fresh water (or a mixture of water and baking soda), then gently rub or brush your teeth and gums for about a minute or so.

Tasty, Tingly Herbal Toothpicks

Cinnamon- or peppermint-flavored toothpicks are often free for the taking at restaurants and are sometimes handed out as samples at health food stores where they're sold. They're tasty and simple to make, and are convenient tools to clean food debris from between your teeth, stimulate your gums, and freshen your breath.

You'll need a half or full box (depending on how many you want to make) of quality wooden toothpicks (round or flat style); a small, lidded glass jar; and enough of your favorite edible essential oil (sweet orange, fennel, anise, peppermint, spearmint, clove, cinnamon bark, tea tree, or tangerine) to cover the toothpicks.

Place the toothpicks either vertically or horizontally in the glass jar, pour in enough essential oil to completely cover them, tighten the lid, and allow them to absorb the essential oil for a couple of days. Next, remove the toothpicks with tweezers and lay them on a plate covered with several layers of paper towels so they can dry for an hour or so. Store them in an airtight glass jar or tin. The leftover essential oil is perfectly good to use again, so don't throw it away!

You can use these toothpicks whenever you want to — just be careful not to stab your gums. Depending on the flavor, they just might satisfy your sweet tooth, too!

HERBAL INFUSION MOUTHWASH

This makes a simple, strong-tasting, highly cooling, mouth-tingling, and refreshing blend. It doubles as a facial astringent for oily, combination, and normal skin, helping to remove excess oil and reduce redness.

2 cups distilled or purified water

2 tablespoons peppermint, spearmint, or rosemary leaves

10 drops tincture of myrrh

RECOMMENDED FOR: *everyone, especially children and those with bad breath or sore or bleeding gums*
USE: *daily*
PREP TIME: *approximately 4 hours*
BLENDING TOOLS: *shake before each use*
STORE IN: *glass or plastic decorative bottle*
YIELD: *approximately 2 cups*

In a small saucepan, boil the water and remove from heat. Add the herb of choice, cover, and steep for about 4 hours.

Strain the liquid, add the myrrh (acts as a mild preservative and antiseptic), and pour into a storage container.

Refrigerate and use within 7 days.

APPLICATION TIPS: Shake bottle immediately before use of approximately 1 tablespoon per mouth rinse. Gargle, then spit it out in the sink (though it will not hurt you if you swallow it).

TO USE AS A FACIAL ASTRINGENT: Saturate a cotton ball or pad and apply to face and throat following cleansing or whenever skin feels oily and in need of freshening.

Natural Breath Fresheners

Even if you carry a spare mini toothbrush and paste in your car, backpack, briefcase, or purse for mid-day freshening, there's no guarantee that a bathroom will always be convenient for brushing. If you ever find yourself in need of fresh breath in a pinch and want to skip the synthetically flavored breath mints and gum, try these tips:

- Swish bottled water in your mouth for 10 seconds and swallow. This helps loosen any food debris and moistens your mouth. A moist mouth harbors less odor-causing bacteria than a dry, pasty mouth.

- Always carry a small, crisp apple within easy reach. After lunch, before a meeting, or whenever you feel the need for a bit of breath cleansing, take a few bites and chew very, very well. This naturally fibrous, juicy, sweet fruit whisks away odor and leaves your mouth feeling wonderfully fresh.

- Chew on a few fennel seeds. They'll leave your breath smelling of fresh licorice. Fennel seeds also relieve gas and upset stomach — two notorious producers of offensive breath.

- After a garlic or onion-laden lunch or dinner out, always make sure to eat that sprig of parsley or watercress sitting on your plate. It's not just a pretty garnish; it really helps eliminate unpleasant lingering food odors and improves digestion.

- Keep handy a small bottle of commercial chlorophyll drops. Chlorophyll is the green pigment found in plants that acts as a natural breath sweetener and digestive aid.

- Buy a small bottle of peppermint, spearmint, or sweet orange essential oil and keep it handy. Apply just one drop to your tongue when your mouth is in need of freshening.

Tincture of Myrrh Mouth Rinse

*M*yrrh has been used for thousands of years as a healing agent for open wounds, an anti-inflammatory, and an astringent. It helps keep gums tight and healthy and treats those that are not.

1 cup distilled water
1 tablespoon tincture of myrrh

RECOMMENDED FOR: *sore gums and teeth, oral infections, and bad breath*
USE: *daily or as needed, up to twice per day*
PREP TIME: *approximately 5 minutes*
BLENDING TOOLS: *shake prior to each use*
STORE IN: *plastic or glass bottle*
YIELD: *approximately 1 heaping cup*

Add both ingredients to a storage container with a tight-fitting lid. Shake well to blend.

No refrigeration is required, but for maximum potency and freshness, please use within 6 months.

APPLICATION TIPS: After shaking the mixture again before using it, pour a tablespoon into a small drinking glass and swish the blend in your mouth for up to 30 seconds (or for as long as tolerated), then spit out in the sink.

FIVE

Natural Care for Glorious Hair

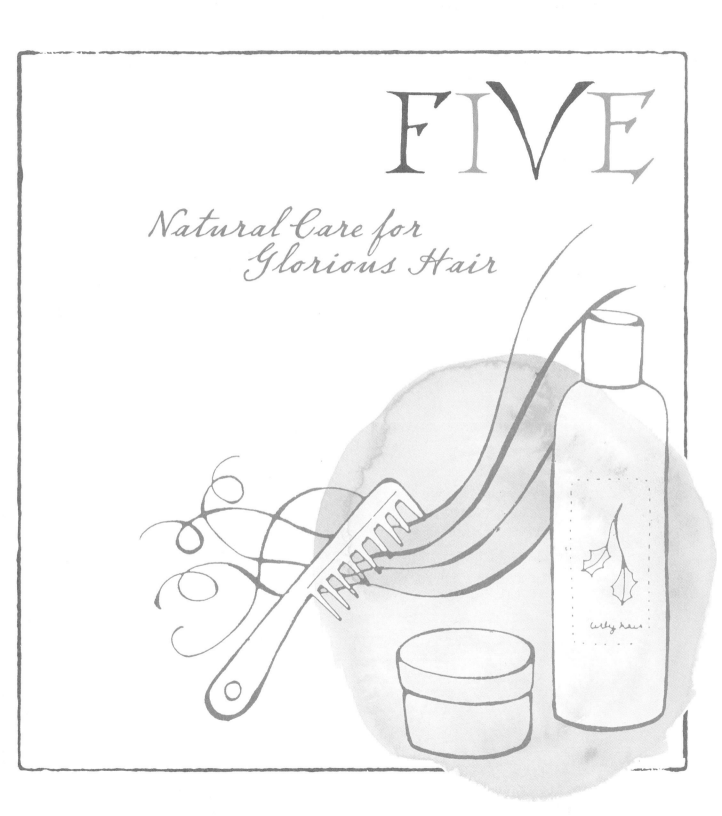

You might say I've had a "bad hair" life: As many children are, I was born relatively bald, and when my hair finally grew in, it was fine, thin, and straight. As if it was a crime, my mother pronounced that it "wouldn't hold a curl."

During the summer just before I entered fourth grade, I had my shoulder-length, light brown, smooth, thin hair shorn into a pixie by my grandmother's hairdresser. I left the shop sporting a tightly roller-curled "do" coated with half a can of lacquer spray. I cried for days.

Sometime in the mid-1970s, when Farrah Fawcett's cascading layers were all the rage, my mother, who usually cut my hair at home, took me to a professional salon to have my now-wavy hair cut like Farrah's. Almost immediately upon cutting my damp locks, unruly curls sprang from my head and the stylist informed me that she'd never be able to achieve the coveted Farrah style on my type of hair. I begged, however, and she finally agreed to cut it but instructed me that I would be a slave to the blow dryer.

I was mortified at what my hair had suddenly become: unmanageable, especially in Georgia's high humidity! In the 1970s, no girl I knew wanted curly hair. Throughout high school I straightened my curly locks chemically and with irons and blow dryers. On low-humidity days, when it remained straight and "beautiful," I smiled with self-confidence, but when it rained and the frizzy curls emerged, I hid, wore a scarf, and cancelled dates.

It wasn't until I was about 23 that I finally met a wonderful stylist with "magic" scissors who thought my hair was naturally beautiful. "It was just cut wrong for its type," he said, and cut my curls so they behaved no matter what the humidity level. In fact, my hair looked better on days when it did rain! I tossed out the blow dryer and clothing iron I used to make my hair flat and allowed my hair to air-dry freely, and all was happy . . . until the gray began to appear in my mid-30s. Little did I know that curly hair becomes kinky hair when it loses its pigment and turns gray. Now in my mid-40s, I have curlier hair than ever, but I'm growing to love it yet again. I'm finally embracing what I've been given.

That's my hair story — but we all have our own version, no matter what type of hair we have: straight, fine, wavy, curly, thick, or thin. In this section you'll learn how to identify and care for the hair you have.

Your Hair Personality

Your hair and its style or natural texture can define you to a degree. Society often deems straight-haired people as the most intelligent, organized, beautiful, and clean-cut. People with wavy hair are thought of the same way, though they are considered to have a bit of a sexy, playful edge, depending upon how their hair is styled. Those with curly or kinky hair often feel compelled to "tame" or smooth their mane in professional circles

ALL HAIR IS FIBER

As the book *Curly Girl* by Lorraine Massey and Deborah Chiel (Workman, 2001) explains, "[t]here isn't much difference chemically between your hair and the fine wool that comes off a pashmina goat." There are at least 100,000 hair fibers on our head, and, like wool, each stretches and absorbs moisture. Because our hair is so much like a fine fiber in our wardrobe, this book suggests that we should care for it as we do a cashmere sweater. Sodium lauryl sulfate or laureth sulfate, detergent ingredients in most shampoos, can also be found in most dishwashing liquids, and while they clean pots and pans in the kitchen by cutting grease, our hair should retain some natural oils. As the authors explain, "stripping them away deprives the hair of necessary moisture and amino acids and makes it look dry and dull."

so it won't be perceived as wild, untidy, or unabashedly sexy.

In fact, as I learned growing up, we have to embrace whatever type of hair we have and care for and style it in ways that flatter and make us feel our best. The three unique hair personalities outlined here each have slightly differing physical structures and thus particular ways in which they prefer to be treated so that they behave their healthy best.

Straight Hair Characteristics and Care

When clean and healthy, the scales of the *cuticle*, or outermost protective layer of each hair strand naturally lie flat, reflecting light that results in high shine. Straight hair swings and is not prone to frizzing. Each strand can be either fine, medium, or coarse in texture and the hair in general can be either oily, normal, or just shy of dry. Straight hair can withstand the most abuse but should still be treated very gently.

Shampooing of straight hair should be limited to a chemical-free cleansing twice per week. On nonshampoo days, use a simple water rinse and a one- to three-minute scalp massage with your favorite hydrating conditioner. This routine will keep your hair and scalp clean and at the same time maintain the natural protective oils on the hair strands.

Wavy Hair Characteristics and Care

Wavy hair can often masquerade as nearly straight during times of low humidity or semicurly and slightly frizzy when humidity is high. The surface scales of the cuticle don't lie quite as flat as those on straight hair, allowing more moisture to penetrate the shaft. This hair tends to shine when healthy and can be fine- or medium-textured (though it's not often coarse). It does tend to be slightly drier than straight hair.

Limit shampooing to a chemical-free cleansing once or twice per week. On nonshampoo days, use a simple water rinse and a one- to three-minute scalp massage with your favorite hydrating conditioner. This routine will keep your hair and scalp clean and at the same time maintain the natural protective oils on the hair strands.

Curly or Kinky Hair Characteristics and Care

As a rule, each strand of curly hair is very fine and fragile, though due to the volume of curls, it may appear that the hair is quite thick or coarse. Actually, curly-haired people have less hair on their head than their straight- and wavy-haired counterparts. This hair type is generally very dry, porous, and brittle, mainly because the natural oils at the scalp have a hard time reaching the ends. Overall, it must be handled with the utmost care. Because the cuticle stands out instead of lying flat, curly hair tends to have less shine. When it's very healthy, however, curly hair can shine and be simply gorgeous.

Abandon the idea that you must shampoo your curls even weekly or monthly. I shampoo only every eight weeks or so and my hair looks and smells wonderful. Here's the trick: Instead of thinking of shampoo, think *moisture*. Shampoo is dehydrating to already dry, curly hair and is simply not necessary for cleansing. Simply perform a

THE ROOT OF THE MATTER

As Mary Beth Janssen explains in her book *Naturally Healthy Hair: Herbal Treatments and Daily Care for Fabulous Hair* (Storey Publishing, 1999), the root of each hair on our head is buried in the dermis and is in direct contact with the bloodstream via capillaries, "any imbalances or toxicity in the body are interpreted and transferred to the hair through the blood supply." I'm sure you've noticed that in times of stress, hormonal fluctuations, illness, and poor diet or when you're exposed to pollutants, your hair registers these challenges much as the rest of your body may.

daily one- to three-minute scalp massage on your wet scalp with a super-hydrating conditioner, followed by a thorough rinsing in the shower to loosen and get rid of excess sweat and sebum. If you follow this regimen, you'll notice more "good hair" days because your hair isn't so dehydrated. Conditioner will become your best friend. If you feel that you must shampoo, then do so only every other week — no more. The recipe for Suds-Free Herbal Hair Wash (see page 304) or any of the herbal rinse recipes in this section make good daily cleansers when you feel the need for a bit more astringency on your scalp.

SIX HEALTHY HAIR HABITS TO START NOW

1. Ditch the stress. Excess stress and worry can cause hair loss and lackluster locks, so meditate, do yoga, take a walk, or enjoy a cup of calming tea.

2. Chill out. Rinse shampoo and conditioner with very cool or cold water to tighten pores, tighten the cuticle, and enhance the shine.

3. Get a trim. Get clipped at the stylist's every eight weeks or so (if you have long hair) or more frequently to maintain the style if you have short hair. Regular trims remove frizzy, split, frayed ends.

4. Cover up. Wear a hat to protect your hair from drying and color-altering sunlight (especially if you have color-treated hair).

5. Minimize heat. Hair fries when dried quickly with a blow dryer set on high, so use the blow dryer only at its lowest setting and, if possible, after hair is already 75 percent air-dried. Keep the use of curling and flat irons to a minimum, too. Heat ruins the health of the cuticle.

6. Balance that diet. Feed your hair with a diet full of hair essentials: protein, biotin (from eggs, organ meats, dried fruit, molasses), iron, iodine, vitamin B12, and omega-3 fatty acids.

Shampoos, Rinses, and Conditioners

The following herbal recipes treat all kinds of hair and many treat the scalp as well. Be sure to look under "Recommended for" in the recipe summary for each recipe to find one that addresses your particular hair characteristics.

BASIC OIL CONDITIONER

This treatment is excellent for dry, abused, sun-damaged, and chemically treated hair. It improves texture and leaves hair soft and silky.

¼ cup more or less (depending on length of hair) of one of the following base oils: extra-virgin olive, jojoba, avocado, or coconut

20 drops lavender, Roman chamomile, rosemary (chemotype verbenon), or basil essential oil

RECOMMENDED FOR: *normal or dry hair*
USE: *once per week*
FOLLOW WITH: *shampoo and light conditioner if desired*
PREP TIME: *approximately 5 minutes*
BLENDING TOOLS: *small bowl and spoon*
STORE IN: *do not store; mix as needed*
YIELD: *1 treatment*

Combine all ingredients in a small glass bowl and stir thoroughly to blend. You can warm the oil if you wish prior to application, but it's not necessary.

APPLICATION TIPS: Apply mixture to dry, clean hair, making sure hair is thoroughly coated. Cover hair with plastic wrap, a plastic food storage bag, or a shower cap, then wrap your head with a warm, damp towel. Replace with another warm towel once the first has cooled. The heat helps the oil to penetrate and condition your hair. Allow the mixture to remain on hair for 30 to 60 minutes. Rinse, then lightly shampoo to remove traces of oil. Follow with conditioner if necessary.

Hair Conditioner and Scalp Stimulator

*T*his formula helps stimulate circulation, encourages hair growth, and aids in balancing sebum production — so don't be afraid to use it if your hair is oily. It has a potent, cooling fragrance and may cause the scalp to slightly tingle. You can actually sleep with this blend on your scalp and hair ends for ultimate conditioning. If your hair and scalp are very dry, you may not need to shampoo afterwards at all.

40 drops rosemary (chemotype verbenon) essential oil
25 drops basil essential oil
20 drops lemon essential oil
15 drops lavender essential oil
15 drops lemongrass essential oil
10 drops peppermint essential oil
½ cup jojoba base oil

RECOMMENDED FOR: *all hair types*
USE: *2 times per week if hair is thinning or dry; otherwise, use once per week*
FOLLOW WITH: *shampoo and light conditioner*
PREP TIME: *approximately 15 minutes, plus 24 hours to synergize*
BLENDING TOOLS: *shake before each use*
STORE IN: *dark glass bottle with dropper top or screw cap*
YIELD: *approximately ½ cup*

Add the essential oils drop by drop directly into a storage bottle. Next, add the jojoba oil. Screw the top on the bottle, wrap your hand around the bottle, and shake the formula vigorously for 2 minutes to blend all ingredients.

Place the bottle in a dark location that's between 60 and 80°F for 24 hours so that the oils can synergize.

No refrigeration is required, but for maximum potency, please use within 2 years.

APPLICATION TIPS: Place 2 teaspoons of the product in a small bowl. Dip fingertips into the mixture and gradually massage the entire amount into your dry scalp for about 3 to 5 minutes, making sure to rub a little onto the ends of your hair. Next, wrap your hair completely with plastic wrap or a shower cap, then wrap it again with a very warm, damp towel. Replace this with another warm towel once it has cooled. Leave on 30 to 45 minutes, then rinse and lightly shampoo your hair. Condition afterward if desired.

Fragrant Hair Sheen

This simple recipe makes hair fragrant and shiny. It also helps to prevent static during cold temperatures and low humidity.

5   drops rosemary (chemotype *verbenon*), lavender, Roman chamomile, or ylang ylang essential oil (or your favorite mix of these)

3   drops castor, coconut, or jojoba base oil (use 6–9 drops if hair is long)

RECOMMENDED FOR: *normal or dry hair*
USE: *after every shampoo or as desired*
PREP TIME: *approximately 5 minutes*
BLENDING TOOLS: *palm of hand*
STORE IN: *do not store; mix as needed*
YIELD: *1 treatment*

Place the drops of the essential oil(s) in the palm of your hand and add the base oil drops.

APPLICATION TIPS: Rub your palms together and gently pat and scrunch your slightly damp hair. Make sure to distribute oils evenly, paying special attention to the ends of hair. If you set your hair, apply this sheen immediately before setting. If you use a blow dryer, apply it in the middle of the styling process.

Suds-Free Herbal Hair Wash

This formula cleanses the hair and scalp without harsh chemicals and foaming agents. These particular herbs nurture the hair follicles and, when massaged into the scalp, lift dirt, debris, and sweat from the scalp and leave a lustrous, glossy condition.

This is an excellent wash for those who have a sensitive scalp, thinning hair, fungus growth, itchy scalp, or dandruff. It also helps to balance a dry or oily scalp. If you exercise often and work up a sweat, this is the perfect "shampoo" to use on a daily basis.

¼   cup bhringaraj, powdered
¼   cup brahmi, powdered (also called gotu kola herb)
¼   cup lavender buds, powdered
¼   cup neem, powdered
Distilled or purified water

RECOMMENDED FOR: *all hair types*
USE: *daily or as desired*
FOLLOW WITH: *conditioner if desired*
PREP TIME: *approximately 10 minutes*
BLENDING TOOLS: *small heatproof ceramic bowl or coffee mug*
STORE IN: *glass or plastic jar, resealable plastic bag, or tin (dry ingredients only)*
YIELD: *1 cup dry ingredients*

Place all dry ingredients in your chosen moistureproof storage container and stir or shake to mix. When ready to shampoo, in a small saucepan boil 1 cup of water and remove from heat. Add to the pan 2 teaspoons of the herb blend or place the herbs in a small heatproof or ceramic bowl or coffee mug and pour boiling water over them.

Cover and allow mixture to steep for 5 minutes, then give the mixture a quick stir to blend. There's no need to strain.

No refrigeration is required for dry ingredients. For maximum potency, please store dry ingredients in a cool, dark, dry area and use within 6 months.

APPLICATION TIPS: Wet hair thoroughly. Pour ½ cup of warm solution (herbs and all) over the top of your head and massage scalp with pads of fingers for 1 or 2 minutes. Rinse. Repeat with remaining solution and rinse well.

HERBAL SHAMPOO FOR ALL HAIR TYPES

*T*his recipe makes an herbal-fragranced shampoo that leaves hair shiny and soft. The mild formula doubles as a face and body wash for all but the driest of skin.

2	cups distilled water
1	tablespoon calendula blossoms
1	tablespoon chamomile flowers
1	tablespoon nettle
2	teaspoons comfrey root
2	teaspoons orange peel
2	teaspoons rosemary
20	drops lavender essential oil
½	teaspoon jojoba base oil (omit if hair is oily)
½	cup natural, chemical-free shampoo base or gentle baby shampoo

RECOMMENDED FOR: *all hair types*
USE: *as needed*
FOLLOW WITH: *your regular conditioner*
PREP TIME: *approximately 45 minutes*
BLENDING TOOLS: *medium-sized bowl, spoon, whisk, strainer*
STORE IN: *glass bottle or plastic squeeze bottle*
YIELD: *approximately 2½ cups*

In a small saucepan, bring the water to a boil and remove from heat. Add the herbs, cover, and allow the mixture to steep for 30 minutes.

Strain the mixture into a medium-sized bowl, add the essential oil and base oil, and stir to blend. Add the shampoo base and stir until thoroughly mixed. Pour into storage container(s).

Refrigerate and use within 4 weeks. If you'd like, you may keep a small bottle in the shower with enough shampoo for about 1 week.

APPLICATION TIPS: Use approximately 1 tablespoon per application. This shampoo will not produce mountains of billowy suds; it doesn't contain strong detergents. It cleans gently with minimal bubbles. Rinse completely with cool water.

Nettle and Sage Oily Scalp Cleanser and Deodorizing Tincture

This tincture freshens, cleanses, and deodorizes an oily scalp or can be used whenever you're in need of a full shampoo but can't seem to find the time. It's perfect to use when hair is styled in cornrow braids and only the scalp needs daily cleansing. It doubles as a facial astringent for oily and combination skin.

¼ cup nettle leaves

¼ cup sage leaves

2½ cups vodka (no added flavors or sweeteners)

RECOMMENDED FOR: *oily or normal scalp*
USE: *daily or as needed*
PREP TIME: *approximately 10 minutes, plus 4 weeks for chemical extraction and tincture formulation*
BLENDING TOOLS: *canning jar, strainer*
STORE IN: *glass jar or bottle*
YIELD: *approximately 2¼ cups*

Place dry herbs in a quart-size canning jar and pour vodka on top of herbs. Cap jar with a piece of plastic wrap, then screw on metal lid. Shake the mixture for about 30 seconds.

Store the jar in a cool, dark place for 4 weeks so that the vodka can extract the valuable chemical components from the herbs. Remember to shake the jar for 15 to 30 seconds each day during the 4-week period.

At the end of the 4 weeks, strain the herbs through a fine strainer, coffee filter, or strainer lined with a piece of hosiery or paper towel. Press or squeeze the herbs to release all the valuable herbal fluid. Pour the liquid into a storage container, then place the container in a dark cabinet.

No refrigeration is required, but for maximum potency, please use within 2 years.

APPLICATION TIPS: Dispense the tincture directly onto the scalp with a plastic or glass eye dropper. Use approximately 1 to 3 full droppers of tincture — enough to cover the entire scalp. Massage into the scalp for 1 or 2 minutes. Use a dark hand towel to blot excess tincture from scalp, and allow to air dry without combing or brushing. *Note:* Avoid getting tincture into eyes; it will sting.

STOP THE STATIC

Try these tips for the prevention of flyaway, dry, static hair:

- Rub 3 to 6 drops of jojoba oil between your palms, then gently finger comb your entire head of hair.
- Apply your favorite natural, spray-on, leave-in conditioner before you style and again lightly after you style your hair.
- Keep hair in good condition by using a weekly hot-oil conditioner.
- Trim dead, split ends at least every eight weeks to prevent snarls, tangles, and unruly hair.
- A bimonthly application of protein- and fat-rich natural mayonnaise on your entire head will help keep hair healthy and shiny and keep the cuticle of each hair smooth, preventing dehydration and flyaways.
- Use a humidifier at home. Hair that is hydrated will lie smooth and not stand on end.

HERBAL SHAMPOO FOR OILY HAIR

*T*his recipe makes a cooling, herbal-fragranced shampoo that leaves hair shiny and soft. It's extremely mild and doubles as a face and body wash for oily, combination, and normal skin.

2	cups distilled water
1	tablespoon lemon balm
1	tablespoon lemongrass
1	tablespoon peppermint
1	tablespoon yarrow
2	teaspoons lemon peel, fresh, chopped (optional)
20	drops lemon, rosemary (chemotype *verbenon*), tea tree, or ylang ylang essential oil
½	cup natural, chemical-free shampoo base or gentle baby shampoo

RECOMMENDED FOR: *oily hair*
USE: *as needed*
FOLLOW WITH: *your regular conditioner*
PREP TIME: *approximately 45 minutes*
BLENDING TOOLS: *medium-sized bowl, strainer, spoon, whisk*
STORE IN: *glass bottle or plastic squeeze bottle*
YIELD: *approximately 2½ cups*

In a small saucepan, bring the water to a boil and remove from heat. Add the herbs and lemon peel (if desired), cover, and allow to steep for 30 minutes.

Strain mixture into a medium-sized bowl, add the essential oil, and stir to blend. Add the shampoo base and gently whisk until thoroughly mixed. Pour into storage container(s).

Refrigerate and use within 4 weeks. If you'd like, you may keep a small bottle in the shower with enough shampoo for about 1 week.

APPLICATION TIPS: Use approximately 1 tablespoon per application. This shampoo will not produce mountains of billowy suds; it doesn't contain strong detergents. Rinse with cool water.

Highlight Boosters

If used several times per week, your hair's natural highlights should begin to appear brighter and more noticeable in about a month or so.

3½ cups distilled water

For blonde hair: sunflower petals, chamomile flowers, lemon rind

For brown/black hair: sage, nettle, rosemary, crushed black walnut hulls

For red hair: calendula blossoms, hibiscus flowers, red clover flowers, rose hips, red rose petals

RECOMMENDED FOR: *Use rosemary, chamomile, sunflower petals, calendula, red clover flowers, red rose petals, and hibiscus flowers on any type of hair. The other herbs are astringent and are best used on hair that is normal or oily.*
USE: *daily or as desired*
FOLLOW WITH: *leave-in conditioner if desired*
PREP TIME: *approximately 45 minutes*
BLENDING TOOLS: *spoon, strainer*
STORE IN: *plastic squeeze bottle*
YIELD: *approximately 3½ cups*

In a small saucepan, bring the water to a boil and remove from heat. Add 5 heaping tablespoons of the herb(s) of your choice, stir, cover, and allow to steep for 30 minutes.

Strain, label, and pour in a storage container.

Refrigerate for 7 days, then discard.

APPLICATION TIPS: Shampoo and condition hair and rinse, or simply wet relatively clean hair. Squeeze out excess water, then generously pour herbal liquid over hair until saturated. Squeeze out excess. Do not rinse. You may follow the rinse with a leave-in conditioner.

Note: Hair that is permed, straightened, or chemically colored is more porous than virgin hair and may not react as you wish. Herbal highlighting liquid will not, however, damage any hair type and offers only temporary subtle highlights and shine. Use dark towels when drying hair; the herbal liquid will stain light-colored ones.

Rinse to Darken Gray Hair

The more porous your hair, the more quickly this rinse will stain the hair strands. Remember, however, this is not a chemical color, so it will not penetrate the hair's cuticle like a semipermanent or permanent color. Thick, coarse hair will be quite resistant to taking any herbal color. Some gray hair may turn light brown, dark blonde, or medium to dark brown. Avoid this rinse if your hair is truly white.

8 cups distilled water

1 cup black walnut hulls, crushed

½ cup nettle

½ cup rosemary

½ cup sage

2 tablespoons regular loose black tea (2 tea bags will do)

¼ cup apple cider vinegar, raw or processed

2 teaspoons jojoba, almond, coconut, or extra-virgin olive base oil

Rubber or latex gloves

RECOMMENDED FOR: *medium to dark gray, light to dark brown, or auburn hair (avoid using on truly white hair); for all hair types except very dry or chemically treated*
USE: *daily for 2 weeks, then every other day or as desired*
FOLLOW WITH: *good-quality leave-in conditioner*
PREP TIME: *approximately 4 hours*
BLENDING TOOLS: *strainer, spoon; shake final product before each use*
STORE IN: *plastic squeeze bottles*
YIELD: *approximately 7 to 8 cups liquid*

In a large pot, bring the water to a boil and remove from heat. Add herbs and vinegar, cover, and steep for 3 to 4 hours. Liquid should be deep brown in color.

Strain and add the base oil. Stir vigorously to blend and pour into storage container(s).

Refrigerate for 2 weeks, then discard.

APPLICATION TIPS: Shampoo as usual or simply wet relatively clean hair. Squeeze excess water, then blot dry. Before you begin this procedure, don your gloves. This rinse will stain hands and nails. Shake bottle thoroughly, apply about ½ to 1 cup of the herbal liquid, and massage into the scalp and hair for about 1 minute. Squeeze out excess and towel dry hair. (Make sure to use a dark towel; this mixture will stain light-colored ones.) Follow with a leave-in conditioner. The more often you use the rinse, the darker the wash of color. This rinse leaves hair remarkably shiny and soft.

You can doctor the mixture with 5 drops each of lavender and rosemary (chemotype *verbenon*) essential oil, if you wish, for added conditioning and fragrance.

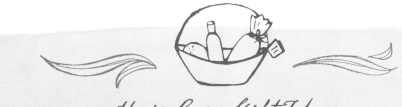

Hair Care Gift Idea

Herbal shampoos and conditioners make great "anytime" gifts for special friends. Any of these recipes can be given in decorative glass or plastic bottles or jars, custom labeled, offering detailed instructions and any necessary expiration dates, and wrapped festively in a decorative wine or gift bag.

Antidandruff Treatments

If you begin to see those pesky white flakes in your hair or on your shoulders, it's best to avoid or at least limit the use of hair gels, sprays, mousses, stiffening balms, hot blow dryers, harsh shampoos, perms, colors, and straighteners. The overuse of any one of these can cause a flaky, dry, irritated scalp, which can imitate dandruff conditions.

True dandruff itches, and can be a result of hormonal disturbances, faulty diet, emotional stress, an increase in sebum production, or a fungal infection. For a very stubborn case of dandruff, consult your health care provider; otherwise, the following recipes work quite well.

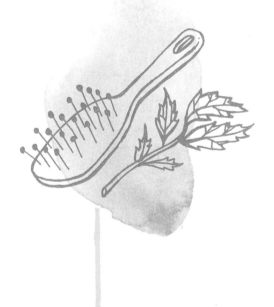

ROSEMARY SOFTENING RINSE

Heady with the heavy, stimulating scent of rosemary, this product gives any hair type luster and body.

4 cups distilled water
½ cup rosemary
1 teaspoon borax

RECOMMENDED FOR: *all hair types, especially lifeless, dull, or flaky hair*
USE: *daily or as desired*
FOLLOW WITH: *Fragrant Hair Sheen (see page 303) if desired*
PREP TIME: *approximately 2 hours*
BLENDING TOOLS: *spoon, strainer*
STORE IN: *plastic squeeze bottles*
YIELD: *approximately 4 cups*

In a medium-sized saucepan, bring the water to a boil and remove from heat. Add the rosemary and the borax, stir, cover, and steep for 2 hours.

Strain and pour into storage bottle(s).

Refrigerate for 7 days, then discard.

APPLICATION TIPS: Use as the final rinse after shampooing or simply conditioning. Do not rinse out. Use approximately ½ to 1 cup per application. Please note that this rinse may stain light-colored towels.

Herbal Vinegar Infusion

ry to use this blend daily until itching and flaking stops. Follow with a natural, leave-in conditioner or detangler if necessary. This slightly medicinal-scented herbal rinse helps to relieve an itchy scalp, remove flakes, and restore your hair's pH balance.

2	cups distilled water
½	cup apple cider vinegar, raw or processed
2	tablespoons rosemary
2	tablespoons sage
1	tablespoon nettle
10	drops tea tree or rosemary (chemotype verbenon) essential oil

RECOMMENDED FOR: *all hair types except very dry*
USE: *daily or as needed*
FOLLOW WITH: *Fragrant Hair Sheen (see page 303) if desired or natural leave-in conditioner*
PREP TIME: *approximately 2 hours*
BLENDING TOOLS: *strainer, spoon*
STORE IN: *plastic squeeze bottle*
YIELD: *approximately 2½ cups*

In a small saucepan, bring the water and vinegar to just shy of boiling. Remove from heat. Add the herbs, cover, and steep for about 2 hours.

Strain, add the essential oil, stir to blend, and pour into a storage container.

No refrigeration is required if used within 2 weeks, or refrigerate for 4 weeks, then discard.

APPLICATION TIPS: Shampoo and condition hair or, if not shampooing, wet hair, condition, rinse, and squeeze out excess water. Shake the bottle vigorously to blend and apply approximately ¼ cup to wet scalp and gently massage for 2 or 3 minutes. Rinse with cool water. *Note:* This rinse may stain light-colored towels.

SIX

In the Mood: Arouse the Senses with Herbal Love Potions

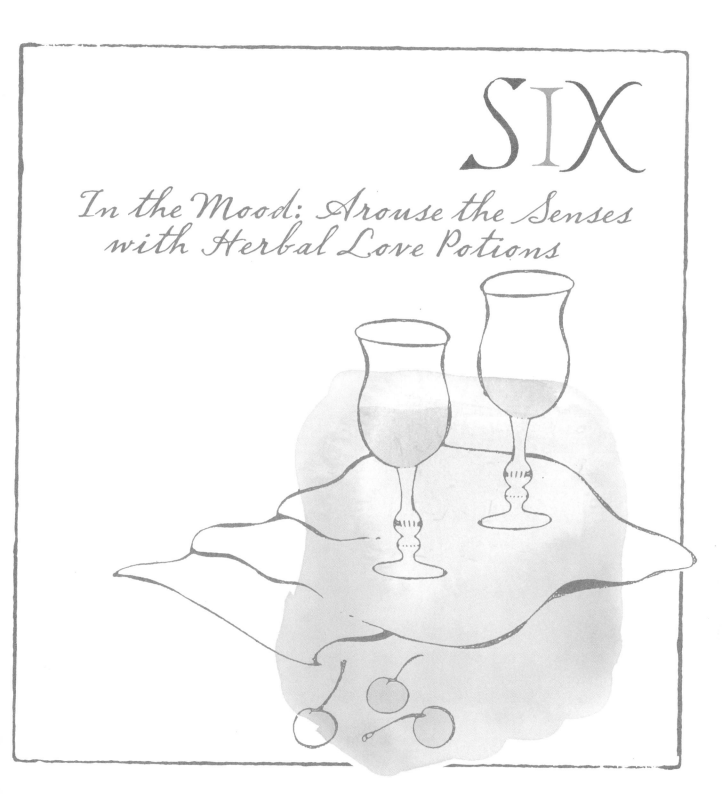

This chapter is written with pure, passionate pleasure in mind! Its recipes offer a bit of a daring departure from the previous topics of skin, hair, and nail care and oral hygiene, but true natural body care extends beyond basic health and aesthetic concerns to include fun; frolic; physical and tactile pleasures; warm, tender sharing; and a celebration of life. The following recipes inspire the spirit of playfulness, spontaneity, relaxation, caring, and creativity. Use these lotions and potions of love to enhance your closest moments and arouse your senses with yummy tastes; soothing textures; fruity, nutty, and erotic aromas; and warming, sweet spices. Here's to a lifelong exploration of delightful and delicious "scentual" and sensual pleasures!

RUBY-RED ROMANTIC APHRODISIAC HERB TEA

T*his red, romantic beverage is perfect for Valentine's Day, Christmas, or any special occasion. It's especially suited for those who wish to abstain from alcohol.*

4 cups distilled or purified water

¼ cup red hibiscus flowers

2 tablespoons lemongrass or lemon balm

2 tablespoons rose hips

Peel of 1 medium orange, preferably organic, cut into slices

Honey, preferably raw

RECOMMENDED FOR: *everyone; even children love it because of its color*
USE: *as desired*
FOLLOW WITH: *an evening of passion*
PREP TIME: *approximately 1 to 2 hours (depending on whether it's served hot or cold)*
BLENDING TOOLS: *spoon, strainer*
STORE IN: *beautiful, medium-sized glass pitcher*
YIELD: *approximately 4 cups*

In a medium-sized saucepan, bring the water to a boil, then remove from heat. Add all ingredients except the honey, cover, and allow the mixture to steep for about 45 minutes until very deep red.

Strain, add the honey to taste, and stir to blend. Pour into your best medium-sized clear or cut-glass pitcher, chill for a couple of hours, and serve. Store refrigerated, covered, for 2 days.

CONSUMPTION TIPS: This round, slightly tart and tasty drink can be served either iced or hot in your most beautiful glasses or cups before, during, or after a light meal. Add fresh orange rind spirals to the pitcher as a colorful and zesty decoration. As an erotic alternative, freeze the tea in ice cube trays to add to mixed drinks, sangria, white wine, ginger ale, or fruit punch.

SIP-'N'-KISS TEA

This tea is sheer sensory delight: It teases and tantalizes, warms and cools, stimulates and tingles. It's perfect as an after-dinner refreshment. This ultimate "kissing beverage" doubles as a comforting gargle for sore throats.

2	cups distilled or purified water
3	peppermint tea bags
1	tablespoon fresh ginger root, grated
2	tablespoons favorite raw honey
1	tablespoon fresh lemon juice

RECOMMENDED FOR: *luscious kissin' and yummy sippin'*
USE: *as desired*
FOLLOW WITH: *lots of lip lockin'*
PREP TIME: *approximately 45 minutes*
BLENDING TOOLS: *mesh strainer, spoon*
STORE IN: *do not store; mix for single use*
YIELD: *approximately 2 cups*

In a small saucepan, bring the water to a boil, then remove from heat. Add the peppermint tea bags and the ginger root and allow the blend to steep for 30 minutes.

Strain the liquid into another pan and add the honey and the lemon juice to taste. Stir to blend. It should taste like a unique mix of home-made lemonade and natural ginger ale with a strong, minty zip.

CONSUMPTION TIPS: Enjoy this zingy tea anytime your mouth needs a bit of refreshing, delicious stimulation. It's wonderful served either over ice or piping hot.

Aphrodite's Lucky-in-Love Liqueur

*T*his love liqueur is gently powerful, warm, spicy, and sweet with a hint of tartness, especially if you add the cherries. Eleuthero is revered for increasing sexual and physical endurance, stamina, energy, and resistance to all types of stress. Spicy, biting ginger has been shown to stimulate circulation and impart warmth to your core, then radiate that heat to the extremities.

½   cup quality, smooth, 80-proof brandy

½   cup quality, smooth, 80-proof vodka, unsweetened

½   cup distilled water

¼   cup favorite raw honey

2   tablespoons eleuthero root (sometimes called Siberian ginseng), dried, sliced or diced

1   tablespoon dried or candied ginger root, diced or sliced (Australian or Thai ginger has the most sumptuous flavor)

½   teaspoon cardamom seeds

5   dried, pitted cherries (optional but a delicious additive)

2   small dried or candied apricots, diced

1   cinnamon stick

1   vanilla bean, cut into ½-inch pieces

RECOMMENDED FOR: *passionate lovers*
USE: *as desired, but avoid if you prefer to abstain from alcohol*
FOLLOW WITH: *an intimate evening, then a good night's sleep*
PREP TIME: *approximately 20 minutes, plus 30 days for extraction process*
BLENDING TOOLS: *shake the storage jar daily*
STORE IN: *decorative glass bottle*
YIELD: *approximately 1¾ cups*

Add all ingredients to a pint-size canning jar or slightly larger glass jar with a tight-fitting lid. Cover the jar with a piece of plastic wrap or a small plastic bag and screw on the lid. Shake the mixture vigorously for 15 seconds to blend the honey.

Store the jar in a cool, dark place for 30 days, remembering to shake the contents daily as the flavors mingle and mellow.

Strain the liquid into a beautiful bottle and cap. You may eat the plumped fruit bits if you wish — but be careful; they're potent!

Refrigerate your love potion and consume within 3 months.

CONSUMPTION TIPS: Pour a small amount of chilled liqueur into two beautiful glasses or goblets. Enjoy this delightful elixir by the sip. Because it can be quite intoxicating, consume just a bit.

Also, try delicately drizzling this nectar onto your lover's body, or drizzle it over sliced, ripe strawberries, peaches, bananas, and cubes of rich pound cake, then seductively feed him or her bites of this decadent dessert.

HEALING AND COOLING LIP BALM AND GLOSS

This luscious lip-treatment recipe doubles as a sweet-flavored, edible, sensual lubricant. It also makes a delightful kissing balm. Note: *This formula is not latex friendly.*

See recipe under Lip Service: Luscious Lips on page 214.
Create the basic formula, but omit the essential oil and lipstick.
APPLICATION TIPS: Apply with wild abandon!

VANILLA VELVET HONEY LIP BALM

Spread this sweet, edible lip-treatment recipe on manicured toes, fingers, and other body parts that yearn to be kissed. Note: *This formula is not latex friendly.*

See recipe under Lip Service: Luscious Lips on page 216.
APPLICATION TIPS: Use your imagination and have a bit of honey-flavored fun!

SMOOTH AND SENSUAL CINNAMON LOVE BALM

T*his soothing, aromatic love balm warms and tingles on contact. A universal favorite, cinnamon's spicy taste and fragrance are enjoyed by both men and women. If you omit the cinnamon flavoring, you can use this balm as a slightly sweet sensual lubricant, or substitute another flavor if cinnamon isn't to your liking. This skin-conditioning formula doubles as a superior lip balm, cuticle softener, and foot cream.*

2 tablespoons plus 1 teaspoon almond base oil

1 tablespoon cocoa butter

1½ teaspoons vegetable glycerin

1 teaspoon beeswax

6–8 drops cinnamon oil flavoring (Follow the package directions for the amount to use for 4 tablespoons of oil-based product.)

RECOMMENDED FOR: *gently warming, spicy lubrication, and tasty kissing*
USE: *as desired*
FOLLOW WITH: *sensual playfulness*
PREP TIME: *approximately 30 minutes, plus 4 hours to set*
BLENDING TOOLS: *small spoon or whisk*
STORE IN: *plastic or glass decorative jar*
YIELD: *approximately 4 tablespoons*

In a small saucepan over low heat or in a double boiler, warm all ingredients except the flavoring until the cocoa butter and beeswax are just melted. Remove from heat and add the cinnamon flavoring. Steadily beat the mixture with a small spoon or whisk for a few minutes until it begins to slightly thicken and become opaque. Pour or spoon into a storage container.

Lightly cover the jar with a paper towel and allow the blend to cool for about 15 minutes before capping. The mixture should sit for 4 hours before use. No refrigeration is required, but for maximum aroma and taste, please use within 6 months.

APPLICATION AND CONSUMPTION TIPS: This formula can be used as a highly emollient, tasty kissing balm, or spread it wherever you need some caressing. It's concentrated, so a fingerful goes a long way! *Note:* This balm is not latex friendly.

Bodacious Body Dessert

This simple combination of coconut oil and vanilla produces a sweet-tasting, slippery, aromatic sensation that is sure to pleasure and please. While experimenting with this recipe, I found myself eating it by the spoonful — it's that good!

3 tablespoons coconut base oil (extra-virgin, unrefined)

1 tablespoon vanilla bean paste, sweetened with sugar

RECOMMENDED FOR: *lovers of rich coconut and vanilla flavors*
USE: *as desired*
FOLLOW WITH: *lots of delicious fun*
PREP TIME: *approximately 10 minutes*
BLENDING TOOLS: *small bowl and spoon*
STORE IN: *small, decorative glass jar*
YIELD: *approximately 4 tablespoons*

Place the coconut oil in a small bowl. Add the vanilla paste and stir or mash the two together to blend.

Note: If the temperature in your kitchen is above 76°F, the mixture will maintain a liquid consistency; if the temperature is below 76°F, it will be a medium-soft solid. Placing the storage container in a shallow pan of hot water for a few minutes before use will quickly soften the oil. Remember, too, that coconut oil melts when it contacts body temperature.

Refrigerate in a pretty jar for 2 months — if it lasts that long!

APPLICATION AND CONSUMPTION TIPS: Spread this edible body dessert anywhere you want to kiss or be kissed. Your skin as well as that of your partner will become slightly sticky and very soft.

Note: This formula is not latex friendly.

BODY HONEY

This edible blend is fabulously tasty, aromatic, and easy to make. It's also comforting to dry skin and works wonderfully well as a hydrating sensual lubricant.

1   teaspoon coconut base oil (extra-virgin, unrefined)

½   teaspoon favorite raw honey

2   drops vanilla, peppermint, cinnamon bark, or sweet orange essential oil (optional)

RECOMMENDED FOR: *sweet kissing and gentle, moisturizing lubrication*
USE: *as desired*
FOLLOW WITH: *sweet pleasure*
PREP TIME: *approximately 3 minutes*
BLENDING TOOLS: *small spoon and small bowl*
STORE IN: *do not store; mix for single use*
YIELD: *1 evening of enjoyment*

In a small bowl, whip together all ingredients. This sweet treat is now ready to use.

Note: If the temperature in your kitchen is above 76°F, the body honey will maintain a liquid consistency; if the temperature is below 76°F, it will be a medium-soft solid.

APPLICATION AND CONSUMPTION TIPS: This body honey is highly spreadable; a little goes a long way. Apply anywhere you desire some slightly sticky, sweet kissing.

Note: This formula is not latex friendly.

TURN UP THE HEAT

James A. Duke, author of *The Green Pharmacy: Anti-Aging Prescriptions* (Rodale, 2001), suggests that if you like hot, spicy ginger (sold in Peruvian markets to heat up even the coldest lover) you can make ginger tea with 1 to 2 teaspoons of freshly grated root per cup of freshly boiled water. Steep the mixture for 10 minutes, then strain it and allow it to cool slightly before drinking.

SEVEN

For Women Only:
Delicate Subjects

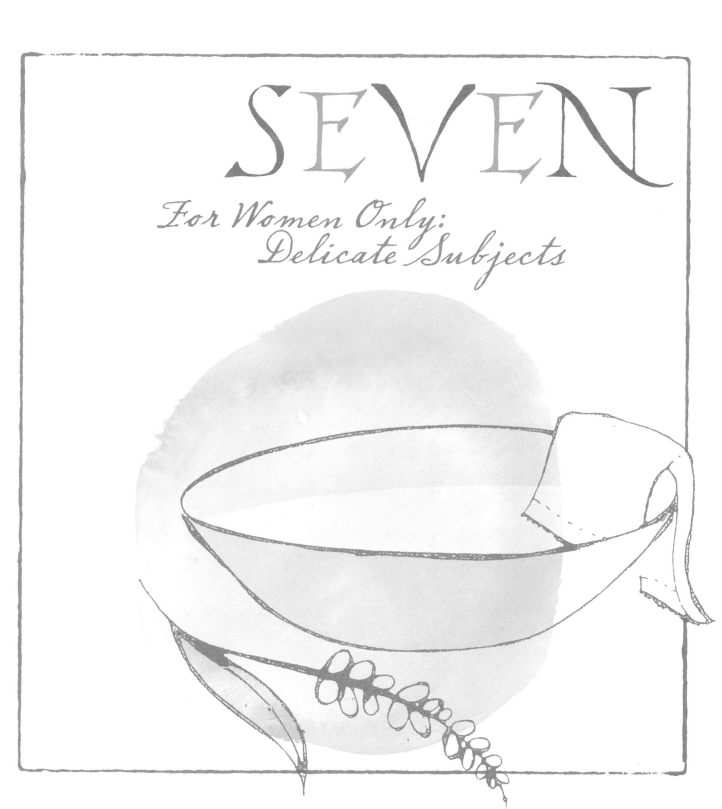

Due to the design and purpose of our bodies, women have unique personal care needs. Unlike men, we menstruate, bear children, lactate, and have feminine hygiene concerns and issues with breast health and vaginal dryness and tenderness. As we age and travel through the various phases of our reproductive cycles, the demands on our bodies change, and with those changes come physical challenges that can often be met with simple, natural, plant-based treatments and preparations. The following recipes were created to help ease women through a few of the more delicate phases of life.

Douches

Most commercial douches are chemical-based (vinegar douches being the exception) and can strip the natural protective pH of the vagina and potentially irritate sensitive tissues. As an alternative, the following recipes are mild and gentle. Keep in mind that these douches are not intended as a substitute for medical treatment, but are instead an aid in relieving minor discomfort. See your health care provider if uncomfortable symptoms arise or persist.

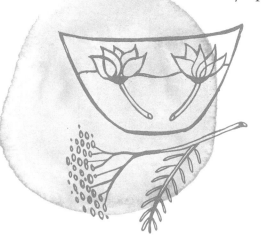

FRESHENING DOUCHE

This recipe makes a slightly astringent, cleansing douche that leaves you feeling fresh. It's perfect to use if you spend your days sitting in snug pants, tights, or panty hose, resulting in an accumulation of sweat and odor or worse, a yeast infection.

2 quarts water, preferably purified and nonchlorinated

4 tablespoons peppermint, rosemary, or yarrow

RECOMMENDED FOR: *general cleansing and freshening*
USE: *once per week*
PREP TIME: *approximately 2 hours*
BLENDING TOOLS: *douche bag, strainer*
STORE IN: *do not store; mix as needed*
YIELD: *1 treatment*

In a medium-sized saucepan, bring the water to a boil, then remove from heat. Add the herb of choice, cover, and steep for about 2 hours.

Strain through hosiery, a paper towel-lined strainer, or a coffee filter to remove all particulate matter, and pour into the douche bag.

APPLICATION TIPS: Proceed as you would normally when douching. Please be sure to thoroughly wash bag, hose, and tip with hot soapy water after use.

COCOA BUTTER VAGINAL LUBRICANT

Cocoa butter, the oily, fragrant part of the cocoa bean, is moisturizing and comforting to dry skin. A small amount (approximately the size of a small marble) inserted into the vagina will quickly melt, adding a soothing slipperiness to dry tissues. It is generally safe to use by all women, even those with sensitivities to ordinary lubricants, and will not contribute to yeast overgrowth. In fact, no natural fatty oil or butter will encourage yeast proliferation unless a sweetener such as sugar, fructose, honey, maple syrup, or molasses is added. Remember, however, that cocoa butter is *not* latex friendly.

Vaginitis Relief

This douche helps to reestablish the naturally acidic pH level in the vagina and leaves behind a comfortable, fresh feeling. I find this recipe especially cooling when tea tree essential oil is included and like to use it just before my period begins, when my abdomen is feeling congested, heavy, and a bit too warm.

2	quarts warm water, preferably purified and nonchlorinated
½	cup apple cider vinegar, raw or refined
10	drops tea tree essential oil (optional)

RECOMMENDED FOR: *external itching and burning; cleans excess vaginal discharge*
USE: *once to 2 times per week (not more often than this)*
PREP TIME: *approximately 5 minutes*
BLENDING TOOLS: *douche bag; shake immediately before use*
STORE IN: *do not store; mix for single use*
YIELD: *1 treatment*

Combine all ingredients in a 2-quart douche bag. Screw in the stopper and give the bag a good shake immediately before use.

APPLICATION TIPS: Proceed as you would normally when douching. See your health care provider if symptoms persist. Please be sure to thoroughly wash bag, hose, and tip with hot soapy water after use.

Love Your Breasts

Because I love myself and I love life, I have my cholesterol and blood pressure checked regularly and schedule my semiannual mammogram along with my annual gynecological visit. You'd think I'd have my longevity health bases covered, right? Wrong! One very important, personal-care step that I admit to skipping is my regular breast self-exams.

Unfortunately, I'm not alone in this regard. An alarming number of women apparently dismiss this vital self-check. One step toward being a healthy, whole woman is to love and take care of yourself first, before reaching out to care for others. When you routinely perform a monthly breast self-exam and massage your breasts on a daily basis, you take breast health into your own hands. With this kind of attention, you're able to recognize any new changes and detect abnormalities as well as support breast health by stimulating circulation and eliminating toxins through the lymph tissues.

Complimentary pamphlets on how to perform a breast self-exam are usually available from your gynecologist, a local women's health clinic or hospital, or from your nearest American Cancer Society. I also found plenty of illustrated instructions on the Internet by simply typing "breast self-exam" in my search engine. Occasionally, I found breast massage techniques as well. You can also search the Web sites of the American Cancer Society (www.cancer.org) or the Susan G. Komen Breast Cancer Foundation (www.komen.org) for further information on breast massage, cancer, prevention, and self-exam techniques.

The following recipes are two of my favorites to use for routine breast massage and general care. The products smell wonderful, are a joy to use, and leave your skin soft and supple.

HERBAL BREAST MASSAGE OIL

This recipe was formulated by herbalist Deb Soule of Avena Botanicals. She grew up in Maine and has been gardening organically for three decades. In 1985 she created the company Avena Botanicals, which offers herbal remedies and body care products made from certified organic and wild-crafted herbs. Deb has authored A Woman's Book of Herbs (Carol, 1998). She also works as a community herbalist, helping clients with various health needs. Avena Botanicals herbal apothecary and gardens are open to the public.

Deb says: "My passion for gardening — working with seeds, moist soil, fragrant flowers, and healing herbs — has inspired me to care for my body in a similar way that I care for the earth. The vibrant colors, soft textures, sensual shapes, and soothing aromas of the herbs growing in my garden delight my senses and restore my spirit throughout the summer. Two favorite herbs, both of which I grow in great abundance for my body care products, are calendula and mugwort. These two herbs infused in a carrier oil are wonderfully effective for easing breast tenderness and improving lymphatic circulation."

If making the infused oils yourself:
Dried organic calendula and
    mugwort flowers and leaves
Organic extra-virgin olive oil

2   tablespoons **each** calendula infused oil and mugwort infused oil

15 drops essential oils: **geranium** to ease breast tenderness and relax the body; **rose** to calm the heart and restore a sense of well-being, trust, and love; a combination of **orange**, **neroli**, and **bergamot** to promote a feeling of emotional harmony and sensual ease; or choose your favorites.

RECOMMENDED FOR: *all women from menstruating age on (do not use bergamot or orange essential oil if pregnant)*
USE: *daily, if desired*
PREP TIME: *approximately 10 minutes if using prepared infused oils or 2 weeks if making the infused oils yourself*
BLENDING TOOLS: *pint jar, cheesecloth (if making the infused oils yourself)*
STORE IN: *glass bottle*
YIELD: *approximately ¼ cup*

TO MAKE AN INFUSED HERBAL OIL: Place ½ cup of dried organic calendula or mugwort flowers and leaves in a clean, glass pint jar. Then add 1 cup of organic extra-virgin olive oil. Cover the jar and place it in a warm window for 2 weeks to allow the herbs to infuse the oil. After this time, pour the oil through unbleached cheese cloth, squeezing as much oil as you can from the herbs.

Keep infused oil in a glass jar in a cool cupboard for up to 18 months.

TO MAKE THE MASSAGE OIL: Pour the infused oils into a 2-ounce glass bottle and add the chosen essential oils from those suggested — just be sure to use no more than 15 drops total of essential oils per 2 tablespoons of carrier oil. Cap and label the bottle and store out of direct light near your bathtub or bed.

No refrigeration is required, but for maximum freshness and potency, please use within 18 months.

APPLICATION TIPS: Shake the infused oil and essential oil blend before using. Regularly massage into the breasts after bathing.

COCONUT OIL — UNIVERSAL SKIN CONDITIONER

Organic, unrefined, extra-virgin coconut oil is used by women the world over as an inexpensive and highly effective body moisturizer. It safely soothes, softens, and lubricates even the most delicate of tissues such as the labia, vagina, and nipples. It takes only a small amount to moisturize, so use it judiciously — and remember that it is *not* latex friendly.

Healing Flowers Beautiful Breasts Salve

I use this formula when performing my monthly breast self-exam: It helps my fingers glide, enabling me to notice any changes with ease. This highly penetrable salve helps rejuvenate, moisturize, and tone breast tissue. This formula doubles as a salve for feet, elbows, lips, and knees and makes a safe belly rub for expectant mothers. Because I love the scent of rosemary and its skin-rejuvenating properties, I occasionally substitute 25 drops of rosemary (chemotype **verbenon***) essential oil for those listed in the recipe.*

5	tablespoons soy bean, almond, or macadamia base oil
2	tablespoons beeswax
1	tablespoon rose hip seed base oil
10	drops neroli essential oil
10	drops ylang ylang essential oil
5	drops rose otto or lavender essential oil

RECOMMENDED FOR: *all women from menstruating age on*
USE: *daily or at least once per week*
PREP TIME: *approximately 15 minutes, plus 20 minutes to cool and set*
BLENDING TOOLS: *small spoon*
STORE IN: *a gorgeous glass jar with a stunning label (though plastic is fine, too)*
YIELD: *approximately ½ cup*

In a small saucepan over low heat or in a double boiler, combine all ingredients except the essential oils and gently warm them until the beeswax has just melted. Remove from heat, allow to cool for 5 minutes, and add the essential oils. Stir to blend.

Pour into storage container(s). Lightly cover with a paper towel and allow to cool for 20 minutes, then cap.

No refrigeration is required, but for maximum freshness and potency, please use within 6 to 12 months.

APPLICATION TIPS: Take a generous fingerful of this salve and rub it vigorously between your palms. Then cup each breast and with your fingertips begin to massage in small circular motions around the outer portion, then repeat around the nipple area. Don't forget to massage a bit of the salve into the décolleté and base of the throat as well.

Pregnancy Stretch Mark Prevention

For most women, pregnancy is a time spent in joyous, life-changing anticipation of the soon-to-arrive precious bundle. Despite the joys, however, those nine months place terrific physical demands on a woman's body — in particular, on her skin — that can be uncomfortable and aesthetically undesirable. These include expansion of the hips, belly, and breasts and the accompanying dryness, itchiness, and tightness and potential for acquiring stretch marks.

What is a stretch mark and how is it formed? Generally curved or wavy, often-times slightly shimmery, at times reddish or pale reddish-purple when new and white or pale silver as they age, stretch marks are stri-ations that appear on the buttocks, breasts, abdo-men, thighs, and occasionally lower back when you gain weight rapidly. Typically, this weight gain is associated with pregnancy, but stretch marks can also develop if you gain only twenty or thirty pounds over a period of a couple of years. I sport a few of these lovely marks and I've neither been pregnant nor more than twenty pounds over my ideal weight. As avid sun worshippers mature, they're prone to stretch marks, too. Stretch marks appear when the skin's subsurface support fibers have broken down, overstretched, and torn. They're generally permanent once they appear, but as a rule they become less noticeable over time.

The key to minimizing the potential for stretch marks, especially during pregnancy, is to take preventive measures before, during, and after your belly (or breasts and buttocks) is in "full bloom" by consistently applying a skin-compatible, topical butter or salve that conditions, hydrates, and comforts the skin. Make a point to apply your product immediately after bathing or showering, and twice more during the day — even after you've given birth! Another tip: Don't forget to hydrate! Be sure to drink plenty of water and caffeine-free herbal teas.

"You're as young as your attitude. If you embrace each stage of life passionately and live abundantly, you will be young forever."

— LYNN J. PARENTINI
AUTHOR, ESTHETICIAN, AND
MASSAGE THERAPIST

BLOOMIN' BELLY BUTTER

This easy-to-make butter is incredibly effective with superior calming and skin-healing properties. It also smells wonderful!

3–4 tablespoons extra-virgin olive, macadamia, avocado, jojoba, sesame, or soybean base oil (Use more for a softer, salvelike consistency.)

1 tablespoon beeswax

20–30 drops lavender essential oil

RECOMMENDED FOR: *pregnant bellies, breasts, buttocks; dry skin; and overweight or rapidly gaining bodies*
USE: *3 times per day or as desired*
PREP TIME: *approximately 15 minutes, plus 20 minutes to cool and set*
BLENDING TOOLS: *small spoon*
STORE IN: *glass or plastic jar or tin*
YIELD: *approximately ¼ cup*

In a small saucepan over low heat or in a double boiler, combine the base oil and beeswax and gently warm until the beeswax has just melted. Remove from heat and add the essential oil. Lavender is a very safe essential oil to use while pregnant, so if you want a potent aroma and greater medicinal value, add 30 drops. Stir to blend.

Pour into a storage container. Lightly cover the container with a paper towel and allow the blend to cool for about 20 minutes, then cap.

No refrigeration is required, but for maximum freshness and potency, please use within 6 to 12 months.

APPLICATION TIPS: Three times per day, apply a generous fingerful to your belly and massage it in completely. Be sure to massage some onto your breasts and buttocks as well.

Rose Hip Restorative Creamy Belly Oil

*R*ose hip seed oil and the essential oils in this recipe are recommended for regenerative skin care, stretch mark prevention, and superior healing of minor cuts and abrasions. All fat–based ingredients are compatible with human sebum and quickly melt into the skin's layers to relieve itchy, stretching skin and provide deep nourishment.

¼ cup jojoba base oil

2 tablespoons rose hip seed base oil

2 tablespoons shea butter, refined or unrefined

10 drops frankincense essential oil (CO_2 extract)

10 drops neroli essential oil

5 drops calendula essential oil (CO_2 extract), if available

RECOMMENDED FOR: *skin before, during, and after pregnancy, during other times of weight gain, and general dry skin complaints*
USE: *3 times per day or as desired*
PREP TIME: *approximately 20 minutes, plus 12 hours to set*
BLENDING TOOLS: *small spoon*
STORE IN: *plastic or glass jar or squeeze bottle*
YIELD: *approximately ½ cup*

In a small saucepan over low heat or in a double boiler, combine all ingredients except the essential oils and gently warm the mixture until the shea butter has just melted. Remove from heat and allow to cool for 10 minutes, then add the essential oils. Stir to blend.

Pour into storage container(s), and cap. The mixture will set to its finished texture in about 12 hours.

Note: You can package the product in a plastic squeeze bottle, but if the formula gets cold, it will become very thick. To return it to a more liquid state, place the bottle in a shallow pan of hot water for a few minutes.

No refrigeration is required, but for maximum freshness and potency, please use within 6 to 12 months.

APPLICATION TIPS: Three times per day, gently massage 1 teaspoon or less of this rich oil into your belly. Be sure to massage some onto your breasts and buttocks as well.

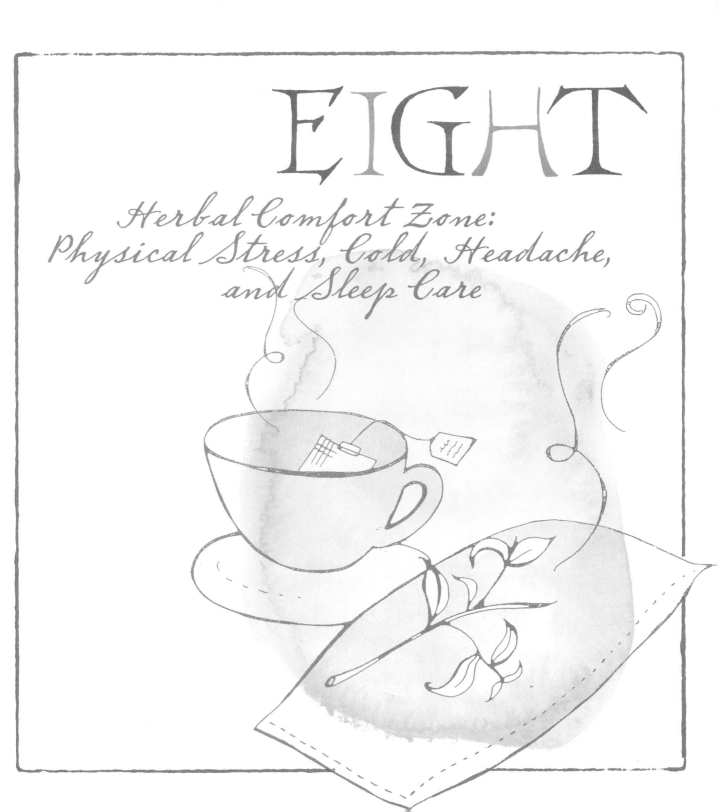

EIGHT

Herbal Comfort Zone:
Physical Stress, Cold, Headache,
and Sleep Care

Every season, every month, every week, even sometimes, every day seems to present its own particular variety of physical distress or discomfort. These annoyances can include the simple aches and pains brought on by the daily grind; the foggy-headedness and misery of a cold or flu bug; the physical or mental exhaustion and accompanying headache brought on by doing too much; or the irritability and lack of focus resulting from too little sleep. It's at these troubling times when herbs in their many forms can offer significant relief and can enhance your well being.

When life deals you a bit of distress and leaves you feeling sick, tired, achy, sleepy, stuffed up, irritable, or simply not feeling quite up to snuff, it's time to put all else aside and take care of yourself. The following recipes will help you feel better, breathe easier, sleep sounder, and even enjoy a deep, peaceful dream or two.

BEAR-OF-A-HEADACHE REFRIGERATOR BALM

If your headache is so intense that you feel as though your head is about to explode, this balm comes to the rescue to help soothe the pain. This recipe doubles as a fragrant, penetrating, softening hand, nail, and cuticle conditioner or foot, knee, and elbow balm for very dry skin. You can leave out the essential oils if you wish.

3   tablespoons shea butter, refined

1   tablespoon jojoba base oil

15 drops **each** of the following essential oils: peppermint; rosemary (chemotype verbenon); Roman chamomile

10 drops lavender essential oil

5   drops sweet marjoram essential oil

RECOMMENDED FOR: *throbbing, pounding, or nervous-tension headaches; insomnia*
USE: *as desired but not more than 3 times per day*
PREP TIME: *approximately 20 minutes, plus 12 hours in refrigerator to firm*
BLENDING TOOLS: *small spoon*
STORE IN: *plastic or glass jar*
YIELD: *approximately ¼ cup or 2 ounces*

In a small saucepan over low heat or in a double boiler, warm the shea butter and the base oil until the shea butter is just melted.

Remove from heat and allow to cool for 10–15 minutes, stirring a few times. Add the essential oils and stir again.

Pour into a storage container and cap. Place it in the refrigerator (or outside if the temperature outdoors is between 35 and 45°F) to harden overnight. The finished product will have a pastelike, buttery consistency.

Note: Once melted, shea butter can remain liquid for many hours, even a couple of days before regaining its semihard texture. Because this recipe contains primarily shea butter, it doesn't thicken into a solid balm if left at a warm room temperature overnight, so I refrigerate it. By morning, the texture is pleasantly firm. I then remove the jar from the refrigerator and allow it to warm to room temperature to get the perfect buttery texture.

No refrigeration is required, but for maximum freshness and potency, please use within 1 year.

APPLICATION TIPS: Massage a small amount of balm wherever your head hurts or you feel painful, muscle tension: temples, forehead, back of neck, or shoulders.

TRANQUILITY IS JUST A WHIFF AWAY

To ease jitters before a speech, calm nervousness and anxiety, cure insomnia, or relieve a pounding headache, simply place a few drops of lavender essential oil onto a tissue and inhale or, alternatively, breathe deeply and deliberately from the lavender essential oil bottle for a few minutes and you should be well on your way to a more peaceful state of mind. Out of lavender? Try Roman chamomile or geranium essential oils; they have similar properties.

OIL OF SUNSHINE: THE ULTIMATE HERBAL COMFORT OIL

This calming oil makes a wonderful face or body moisturizer and bath oil for all skin types except oily skin, and it's perfect for infants with diaper rash. It can be used to help heal minor skin irritations, to relieve muscle pain, and to ease a young, active child before bedtime. I make a large batch every year from fresh picked flowers harvested from my garden. It's one of my favorites!

3 parts chamomile flowers, fresh or dried

1 part lavender buds, fresh or dried

Extra-virgin olive oil (enough to completely cover flowers)

25 drops lavender essential oil

15 drops German chamomile essential oil

15 drops Roman chamomile essential oil

1 quart-size canning jar, sterilized

RECOMMENDED FOR: *anyone with headaches, sore muscles, insomnia, skin irritations, eczema, psoriasis, bug bites, or dry skin*
USE: *as desired*
PREP TIME: *approximately 1 month to infuse, plus a short amount of set up and bottling time*
BLENDING TOOLS: *quart-size canning jar, knife or chopstick, spoon, strainer, funnel*
STORE IN: *glass or plastic bottles*
YIELD: *approximately 3 cups (depending on whether flowers are fresh or dried, how tightly packed in the jar, and the size of flower heads)*

FRESH FLOWER PREPARATION (OPTIONAL): If you want to use fresh flowers (which I highly recommend) and have access to them at peak blossoming time, harvest a total quantity of 5 or 6 cups in the morning before the sun gets too warm and after the dew has just dried.

Spread the flowers (and their bits of attached greenery) onto a clean screen, pillow case, or long strip of paper towels in a warm location where its barely breezy or calm and mostly shady. The area should also be protected from wafting animal dander, dust, and flies. I dry my flowers on a table in my study or on the back seat of my car.

Allow the flowers to wilt and partially dry for 36 to 48 hours. If humidity is very high, add another 24 hours to this time. This process should remove sufficient moisture from the flowers so that mold and bacterial growth will not be introduced into your infused oil.

OIL PREPARATION: Loosely fill a dry, clean quart-size canning jar with the wilted or dried flowers (they should reach to within an inch or so of the top of the jar).

Drizzle the olive oil over the flowers until it has reached the bottom of the jar and has completely covered the plants at the top. The flowers will settle with the weight of the oil, so don't worry if it looks as though you don't have enough flowers in the jar. Make sure all plant matter is submerged and none is exposed to air. The jar should be quite full of oil and herbs. There shouldn't be more than 1 inch of air space between the contents and the lid. Add more oil if necessary to bring contents up the this level.

After you've added all the oil, stick a clean knife or chopstick into the jar and gently stir to remove any trapped air bubbles.

BLEND AND INFUSE: Place a piece of plastic wrap or small plastic bag over the mouth of the jar (to avoid having the metal jar lid contacting the herbs) and tightly screw on the lid. Shake the jar several times to blend the herbs and oil thoroughly.

Place the jar in a warm, sunny location such as a south-facing window sill and allow the flowers to solar infuse for 1 month. Shake the jar for 30 seconds or so daily.

After this time, carefully strain the oil through a fine strainer, then strain again through muslin, a bit of hosiery, or (easiest and my preference) your strainer lined with a coffee filter to remove all debris. Squeeze herbs to extract all of the oil. Next, add the essential oils and stir well to blend.

PACKAGE: Pour the finished oil into several storage containers (a funnel comes in handy for this) and store.

Note: If mold forms in your jar during the 30 days of infusion, you'll need to discard the product and begin again. Prior to infusing herbs in oil, always make sure the jar is sterilized and thoroughly dry and (if you're using fresh herbs as opposed to dried) that they're limp and wilted and haven't been exposed to mist, fog, or extremely high humidity.

No refrigeration is required if used within 6 months, or refrigerate for up to 1 year, then discard.

APPLICATION TIPS: To help heal skin irritations and bug bites: Apply as desired. To relieve muscle strain and pain and headache: Massage into affected areas. To ease an active child before bedtime: Apply as a chest rub; the combination of your touch along with the gentle sedative properties of the formula will lull a child into dreamland.

HERBAL DECONGESTING STEAM

This herbal steam may be used regularly by everyone except those with weepy acne or acne rosacea; those suffering from very sensitive, sunburned, or windburned skin; those who have broken capillaries; and those suffering from asthma. Steam heat can further irritate these conditions.

3–4	cups distilled or purified water
2	teaspoons peppermint or eucalyptus leaves
1	teaspoon comfrey or marsh mallow root
1	teaspoon rosemary leaves
1	teaspoon thyme leaves

RECOMMENDED FOR: *all cold, flu, and sinusitis symptoms*
USE: *daily, but not more than 5 days in a row as skin could become irritated, but use your own judgment*
FOLLOW WITH: *a few dabs of Bee Clear Sinus Vapor Balm (page 342)*
PREP TIME: *approximately 10–15 minutes*
STORE IN: *do not store; mix as needed*
YIELD: *1 treatment*

In a medium-sized saucepan, bring water to a boil. Remove from heat and add the herbs, cover, and steep for 5 minutes. Place the pan of infused herbs in a safe, stable place where you can sit comfortably for 10 minutes.

If you'd like to make up a larger batch of herbs to have handy for yourself or a needy friend or relative, store the dry ingredients in an air-tight zip-seal plastic bag, plastic or glass jar, or tin, and keep in a dark, dry, cool place.

No refrigeration is required for dry ingredients, but for maximum freshness and potency, please use within 6 months to 1 year.

APPLICATION TIPS: Remove the cover from the pan. Drape a large bath towel over your head and shoulders and the steaming herbs to create a tent. With your eyes closed and your face 10 to 12 inches from the edge of the pot (to avoid burning your skin and lungs), breathe deeply and relax as you allow the steam to reach deep into the sinus cavities, lungs, and throat.

This procedure follows the same steps as those for an herbal facial steam, so begin with clean skin. Follow the steam with a splash of lukewarm water and your favorite facial toner or astringent and moisturizer. Don't forget to apply a dab of Bee Clear Sinus Vapor Balm (page 342) under your nose, on your throat, chest, temples, or anywhere the vapors might help you breathe easier.

Bee Clear Sinus Vapor Balm

This formula is designed to help relieve nasal congestion due to hay fever, upper respiratory allergies, common cold, flu, or sinusitis. The vapors contain antibacterial and antiviral properties to aid in healing the source of your stuffiness, shrink swollen mucous membranes, and alleviate tightness in your chest. I love the fragrance so much that I also use it as a soothing headache-relief balm. This recipe doubles as a hand, foot, nail, and lip balm to soothe and soften dry skin.

- 5 tablespoons soybean base oil
- 1 tablespoon beeswax
- 1 tablespoon cocoa butter
- 1 tablespoon shea butter
- 25 drops cajeput essential oil
- 20 drops eucalyptus radiata essential oil
- 10 drops **each** of the following essential oils: lavender; peppermint; balsam fir; sweet birch
- 5 drops tea tree essential oil
- 5 drops thyme (chemotype *linalol*) essential oil
- 2 drops clove essential oil

RECOMMENDED FOR: *stuffy sinuses, general respiratory congestion*
USE: *as desired*
PREP TIME: *approximately 30 minutes, plus 12 hours to completely set*
BLENDING TOOLS: *small spoon*
STORE IN: *plastic or glass jar or tin*
YIELD: *approximately ½ cup or 4 ounces*

In a small saucepan over low heat or in a double boiler, combine all ingredients except the essential oils and gently warm them until all solids are just melted. Remove from heat. Stir a few times to blend the mixture thoroughly, and then allow it to cool for 5 minutes. Add the essential oils and stir again.

Pour into storage container(s), lightly cover with a paper towel, and allow the blend to cool for 15 minutes, then cap. Allow the balm to harden overnight at room temperature.

Note: Because both cocoa butter and shea butter are included, the balm may continue to change texture slightly for another 24 hours.

No refrigeration is required, but for maximum freshness and potency, please use within 1 year.

APPLICATION TIPS: Spread a bit of balm under the nose, on the throat, on temples, chest, back, or even on the soles of the feet.

"TO SLEEP PERCHANCE TO DREAM" BALM

This balm is absolute heaven! You can't help but be lured into dreamland when you take a deep whiff of this citrus-floral dream enhancer. These essential oils are said to open channels for peaceful dreaming and creative visualization while aiding in the relaxation of mind and body. I also like to use this balm to help relieve headaches or neck or shoulder tension, or when I am feeling anxious or irritable. With or without the essential oils, it also performs wonderfully as a hand, foot, nail, and lip balm.

5	tablespoons soybean base oil
1	tablespoon beeswax
1	tablespoon cocoa butter
1	tablespoon shea butter
20	drops sweet orange essential oil
20	drops tangerine essential oil
15	drops geranium essential oil
15	drops lavender essential oil
10	drops neroli essential oil
5	drops vanilla essential oil (optional)
4	drops rose otto essential oil (optional)

RECOMMENDED FOR: *insomniacs; encouraging peaceful, creative dreams; relieving muscular tension and headaches; calming irritable children over 2 years of age*
USE: *as desired*
PREP TIME: *approximately 30 minutes, plus 12 hours to completely harden*
BLENDING TOOLS: *small spoon*
STORE IN: *plastic or glass jar or tin*
YIELD: *approximately ½ cup or 4 ounces*

In a small saucepan over low heat or in a double boiler, combine all ingredients except the essential oils and gently warm until all solids are just melted. Remove from heat. Stir a few times to blend the mixture thoroughly, and then allow it to cool for 5 minutes. Add the essential oils and stir again.

Pour into storage container(s). Lightly cover them with a paper towel and allow the blend to cool for 15 minutes, then cap. Allow the balm to harden overnight at room temperature. Because both cocoa butter and shea butter are included, the balm may continue to slightly change texture slightly for another 24 hours.

Note: This formula contains highly volatile citrus oils. Their scent and healing properties evaporate more rapidly than those of other essential oils, resulting in a shorter shelf life than most of the balms and salves included here. While the balm itself will last for over a year, the aroma will diminish significantly.

No refrigeration is required, but for maximum freshness and potency, please use within 6 to 8 months.

APPLICATION TIPS: Spread a bit of balm under the nose, on the throat, temples, chest, back, or even on the soles of your feet. Inhale deeply and feel blissfully Zen-like.

Sandman Blissful Sleep Balm

*T*his soothing balm will transport you to a calmer, more peaceful place. In making it, you can substitute the infused oil from Oil of Sunshine (see page 338) for the olive and castor base oils. Its strong chamomile aroma will almost overtake the essential oil fragrances, but it won't diminish their properties. You'll enjoy its fresh, earthy, green, floral scent.

2	tablespoons plus 1 teaspoon extra-virgin olive base oil
1	tablespoon castor base oil
2	teaspoons beeswax
20	drops bergamot essential oil (substitute sweet orange essential oil if making this formula for children 2 years of age and under)
10	drops grapefruit essential oil
5	drops **each** of the following essential oils: sweet marjoram; ginger; rosemary (chemotype *verbenon*); lavender; balsam fir

RECOMMENDED FOR: *insomniacs of all ages and those suffering from nervous tension, anxiety, headaches*
USE: *as desired*
PREP TIME: *approximately 15 minutes, plus 15 minutes to set*
BLENDING TOOLS: *small spoon, fork or chopstick*
STORE IN: *plastic or glass jar or tin*
YIELD: *approximately ¼ cup or 2 ounces*

In a small saucepan over low heat or in a double boiler, warm the base oils and the beeswax until the wax is just melted. Remove from heat and stir the mixture a few times to blend. Add the essential oils directly to storage container, then slowly pour into the container the oil/wax mixture. Gently stir the balm with a fork or chopstick to blend.

APPLICATION TIPS: Simply rub a bit of balm under the nose, on the throat, temples, hands, or chest (or all five places) just before bedtime or whenever you're suffering from a headache, nervous tension, or anxiety. Inhale deeply and drift into a scented sleep.

Rub Out the Ache Herbal Creamy Compound Oil

*T*he essential oils in this herbal compound are specifics for relieving inflammation, pain, and bruising. Combined with massage, this formula will increase circulation to the injured or sore area and aid in rapid improvement. The coconut oil and shea butter in the mixture make this remedy highly penetrable: It's quickly absorbed and relaxes injured tissues.

2   tablespoons soybean, almond, macadamia, or extra-virgin olive base oil

1   tablespoon coconut base oil (extra-virgin; unrefined)

1   tablespoon shea butter, refined (*Note:* Unrefined will work, but its fragrance will mask the aroma, though not the properties of the essential oils.)

20   drops sweet birch essential oil

15   drops eucalyptus radiata essential oil

10   drops helichrysum essential oil

10   drops rosemary (chemotype *verbenon*) essential oil

5   drops German chamomile essential oil

RECOMMENDED FOR: *bruises, general aches and pains, sore feet, arthritis, stiff muscles, headaches, bug bites, stuffy sinuses*
USE: *as desired, but not more than 3 times per day*
PREP TIME: *approximately 30 minutes, plus overnight to set up and slightly thicken*
BLENDING TOOLS: *small spoon; shake before each use*
STORE IN: *plastic squeeze bottle*
YIELD: *approximately ¼ cup or 2 ounces*

In a small saucepan over low heat or in a double boiler, warm all ingredients except the essential oils until the coconut oil and shea butter are just melted. Remove from heat and allow the blend to cool for 10–15 minutes, stirring a few times.

Add the essential oils directly to a storage container. Pour the oil/butter mixture into the storage container. Cap and shake well.

Note: Due to the inclusion of shea butter, this formula will not reach its final opaque, creamy oil consistency for 12 hours. I usually let my bottle rest on the counter overnight and in the morning, once

I shake it vigorously, it's ready to use. If the mixture is exposed to cool temperatures (50 to 60°F), it will get quite thick. If this happens, simply place the bottle in a shallow pan of hot water for 5 minutes to soften the blend. No refrigeration is required, but for maximum potency and freshness, please use within 6 to 12 months.

APPLICATION TIPS: This is a true multi-use formula: Apply a few drops to temples to relieve headaches, directly to injured muscles to prevent bruising, to strained or tight muscles to release tension, to arthritic joints to free movement, or to sore feet to ease pain. I apply a drop to bug bites (it seems to alleviate the sting) and rub it into my chest when I feel a cold coming on or I'm seasonally stuffy and wheezy.

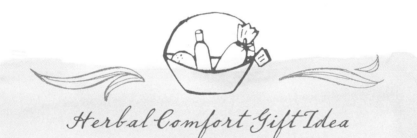

Herbal Comfort Gift Idea

The first recipe in this chapter, Oil of Sunshine, makes a marvelous, fragrant, healing gift for anyone who lives a frazzled life. This is truly a blessed oil — an offering from your heart to a friend or family member in need.

- Present this formula in a cobalt blue or green glass bottle or (because it has such a gorgeous, yellow-green color) in a clear bottle.
- Hand paint or stencil a label and attach instructions for use.
- For a more grand gesture of good will and good health, create a gift basket of solace or a gift basket of renewal and restoration by combining this oil with an herbal eye pillow, dream pillow, and sleep balm.

FORTY WINKS HERBAL EYE PILLOW

*E*ye pillows are a must for me if I'm sleeping in a room where I can't completely block out all light or if I'm napping during the day. Many people find the light weight or pressure of the pillow on the eyes to be sedating. The herbs in this recipe combine two relaxing florals with the sharpness of mint, but you can experiment with other herbs as long as they aren't too stimulating.

1   rounded ½ cup whole flax seeds
1   rounded ½ cup lavender buds
1   rounded ½ cup peppermint leaves
1   rounded ½ cup crushed rose petals
10 drops lavender essential oil
5   drops peppermint or rose otto essential oil

RECOMMENDED FOR: *insomniacs and those in need of darkness to sleep*
USE: *anytime*
PREP TIME: *approximately 30 to 45 minutes*
BLENDING TOOLS: *medium bowl, large spoon*
STORE IN: *zip-seal plastic bag*
YIELD: *1 eye pillow*

TO MAKE THE PILLOW: Choose a fabric that's aesthetically pleasing to you and soft to the touch, such as silk, satin, flannel, or velveteen. My favorite size for an eye pillow is approximately 4 inches wide by 10½ inches long. When you cut your two fabric rectangles for the pillow, allow for a ½-inch hem all the way around. The rectangles should be 5 inches wide by 11½ inches long. Put the fabric together with right sides facing, hem three sides (leaving a narrow end open for stuffing), and turn the pillow case right side out.

As a quick alternative to cutting and measuring fabric and taking out the sewing machine, if you happen to have an old silk, satin, flannel, fine-wale corduroy, or brushed cotton long-sleeved blouse on hand, an 11-inch to 12-inch length of sleeve will work. It's easy to adjust the amount of herbal "stuffing" to suit the size of the sleeve.

TO MAKE THE "STUFFING": Place all the ingredients except the essential oils in a medium-sized bowl and stir to blend the mixture. Add the essential oils drop by drop and continue slowly stirring. Spoon the mixture into the narrow end of your pillow casing or sleeve. You don't want to stuff the eye pillow until it is full and tight. It should remain somewhat floppy so that when it's placed over your eyes and the bridge of your nose, it will comfortably conform to your face. After you've filled the case, tuck the raw edges inside and hem the end closed by hand.

No refrigeration is required, but to prolong the herbal properties and keep the flax seeds from becoming rancid, please store your pillow in a cool cupboard or drawer and in a zip-seal bag. It will provide up to 6 months of effective comfort.

APPLICATION TIPS: Gently place the eye pillow over both eyes and the bridge of your nose, breathe deep, and go to sleep. If your bedroom is particularly warm or you're experiencing a headache, chill the pillow in the freezer for 30 minutes before applying it. The cool relief it provides is amazing.

OF CATS AND DREAM PILLOWS

Whenever I use one of these pretty pillows and forget to put it away in the morning, I frequently find it in the paws of my big, male, Maine coon cat. Come time for his midafternoon nap, I find that he's claimed it for his own and, completely zonked, is wrapped around it, snug as a bug. Time to make myself a new one . . . again.

If you're a cat owner, be careful where you leave your little pillow. Your furry friend might want to steal a bit of sleep comfort in hopes of mice dreams.

Dream Maker Herbal Sleep Pillow

Herbal dream or sleep pillows have been used by children and adults for centuries to induce relaxation and melt away the day's nervous tension. The delicate scent is said to bring on pleasant dreams.

¼ cup chamomile flowers

¼ cup lavender buds

¼ cup lemon balm leaves

¼ cup rose petals

⅛ cup hops

2–3 drops lavender, Roman chamomile, geranium, or neroli essential oil

I 3- by 5-inch muslin drawstring bag or decorative, soft fabric pouch

RECOMMENDED FOR: *insomniacs in need of deep sleep and sweet dreams*
USE: *daily if you wish*
PREP TIME: *approximately 10 minutes (if you use a premade muslin drawstring bag)*
BLENDING TOOLS: *medium-sized bowl, spoon*
STORE IN: *3- by 5-inch muslin drawstring bag or custom-made pouch; store pillow in nightstand*
YIELD: *1 dream pillow*

Place all the herbs in a medium-sized bowl and stir to blend. Add the essential oil and stir a few more times. Loosely stuff your pouch with the herb mixture and tie it or sew it tightly. If you make your own pouch, fabrics such as flannel, sand-washed silk, satin, velveteen, and brushed cotton are soft and inviting. A dream pillow has a relatively short shelf life because the herbs are exposed to air. The scent lasts for a couple of months if you store the pillow in a nightstand, away from heat and light.

Note: The amounts of herbs listed are a close approximation of what you'll need and can vary depending on the size of plant materials and your particular pouch size. Don't pack your pillow so tightly that the herbs can't breathe and move.

APPLICATION TIPS: Simply tuck your fragrant pouch into your pillowcase right before going to sleep, or do as I do and hold it close to your face. Breathe deeply and drift off.

NINE

Bugs Be Gone:
Natural Insect Repellents

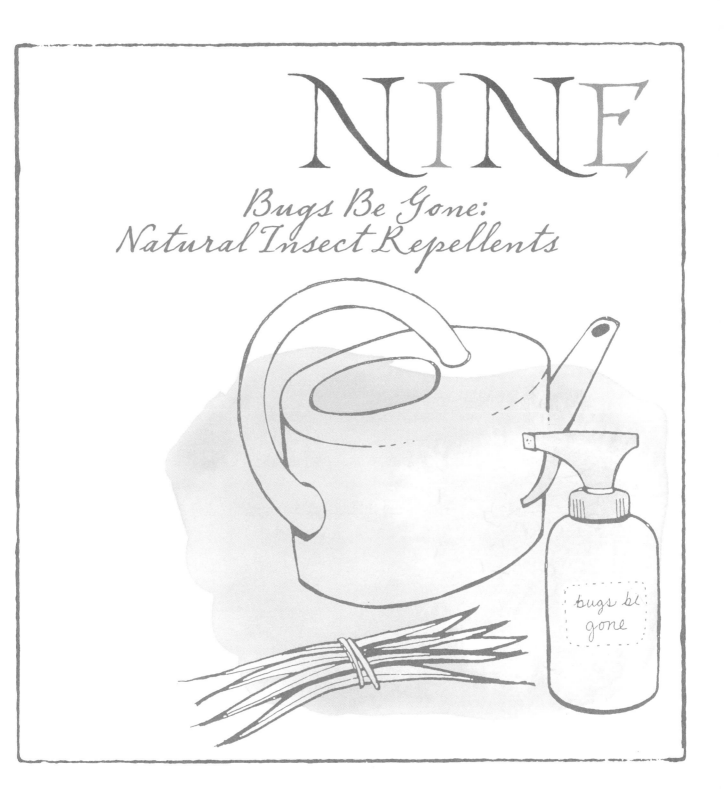

bugs be
gone

Most insect repellents on the market today are full of chemicals and replete with unpleasant, toxic aromas that are often masked by irritating synthetic fragrances. Why would you want to repeatedly spray your body with unhealthful products in order to enjoy the outdoors? Many people, myself included, are highly sensitive or even allergic to the chemicals in these commercial products.

Thank goodness there are now a handful of truly nontoxic insect repellents available commercially from health food stores or online in case you don't want to make your own formula at home. If you do want to craft your own antibug material, the following easy-to-create, aromatic recipes offer natural alternatives to chemical-based sprays. These formulas tend to work best on days when the mosquitoes, no-see-ums, deer flies, black flies, midges and other local nasties are only slightly to moderately hungry. If they're voracious, additional protection such as a net hat, net body suit, or just a high-collared shirt and lightweight pants can come in handy.

Note: Prior to venturing outdoors, always remember to avoid wearing any type of fragrance (aside from your insect repellent), including cologne, aftershave, scented deodorant, shampoo, conditioner, body lotion, breath

REASONS NOT TO USE A CHEMICAL-BASED MOSQUITO REPELLENT

Read some of the precautionary statements — in tiny print — on the labels of popular, commercially available chemical-based mosquito repellent sprays. Perhaps you'll think twice in the next bug season before using this type of product on your skin and seek natural, nontoxic alternatives and cover up with clothing and hats when necessary.

mints, hair gel, bath oil, soap, or even laundry detergent and linen sprays. Biting insects seem to be attracted to the same scents that we like.

"Fend Off" Herbal Oil Insect Repellent

I make sure to use this oil every day when bugs are at their worst — and sometimes twice per day to achieve the effect of literally saturating my pores with it's bug-repellent properties. As a bonus, my skin is very soft and conditioned — and occasionally I even get a compliment on my unusual fresh "perfume." If they only knew!

½ cup soybean base oil (*Note:* This oil has natural bug-repellant properties.)

15 drops **each** of the following essential oils: lemongrass; geranium; catnip

10 drops basil or eucalyptus radiata essential oil

RECOMMENDED FOR: *all skin types except very oily*
USE: *as needed*
PREP TIME: *approximately 10 minutes, plus 1 hour to synergize*
BLENDING TOOLS: *shake container before each use*
STORE IN: *plastic or glass spritzer, pump, or squeeze bottle*
YIELD: *approximately ½ cup or 4 ounces*

Add all ingredients directly to a storage container. Shake the mixture vigorously to blend.

Allow the oil to synergize, for 1 hour.

No refrigeration is required, but for maximum bug-repelling freshness and potency, please use within 6 to 12 months.

APPLICATION TIPS: I like to apply this formula onto my palms first, then massage the oil into areas that need bug protection. During the height of bug season, when the little biters are on their worst behavior, I actually use this pleasantly fragranced, oil-based repellent as an after-shower massage oil, bath oil, hair conditioner, scalp massage oil, and all-purpose body moisturizing oil.

Bite-Me-Not Balm

*T*his formula has a woodsy, somewhat nutty, earthy herbal aroma that is generally pleasing to everyone. It doubles as a basic conditioning, moisturizing, all-purpose body balm if you leave out the essential oils.

3 tablespoons soybean base oil (*Note:* This oil has natural bug-repellant properties.)

1 tablespoon neem base oil

1 tablespoon beeswax

20 drops catnip essential oil

10 drops **each** of the following essential oils: lemongrass; rosemary (chemotype *verbenon*); thyme (chemotype *linalol*)

5 drops cedar essential oil

RECOMMENDED FOR: *all skin types*
USE: *as needed*
PREP TIME: *approximately 15 to 20 minutes, plus 1 hour to set and synergize*
BLENDING TOOLS: *small spoon*
STORE IN: *plastic or glass jar or tin*
YIELD: *approximately 5 tablespoons or ⅓ cup*

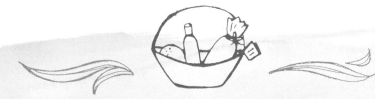

Insect Repellent Gift Idea

What better gift to give the outdoors enthusiast, gardener, hiker, hunter, fisherman, bird watcher, neighborhood jogger, or dog walker in your life than a bottle of your chemical-free, fragrant, effective insect repellent?

• Create one of these easy-to-make recipes.

• Attach a cute, handmade, simply illustrated label with a catchy name such as "Bug Busters" or "Bug Me Not."

• Include complete instructions for use.

In a small saucepan over low heat or in a double boiler, warm the base oils and the beeswax until the wax is just melted. Stir the mixture gently a few times. Remove from heat and allow the blend to cool for 5 minutes. Add the essential oils and stir a few more times.

Pour into storage container(s) and cap. Allow the balm to set and synergize, for 1 hour. I like to store this formula in several small containers that I can keep in my car, my purse, the bathroom, my backpack, or wherever I might need some bug protection.

No refrigeration is required, but for maximum freshness and potency, please use within 1 year.

APPLICATION TIPS: You can actually massage this balm all over your entire body, but I prefer to dab a little on my temples, neck, wrists, chest, waistline, and ankles or, in other words, on the entry points that bugs use to fly or crawl into my clothing.

ITCH AND STING RELIEF

Insects may be small, but their bites can deliver a big dose of itchy, inflamed misery! To counteract this discomfort, there are many natural remedies that work amazingly well.

- Apply a simple baking soda and water paste directly to bites and leave on for at least an hour.
- For an anti-itch bath, add ½ to 1 cup baking soda to running luke-warm water and soak for 15 to 20 minutes.
- Apply a drop of lavender or tea tree essential oil directly onto each bite to reduce inflammation and help prevent infection.
- Make a solution of 1 part apple cider vinegar to 3 parts water, and rinse the irritated area. Repeat this procedure several times until the itching decreases in intensity.
- Apply a drop of neem base oil to each bite. Neem is a naturally cooling oil with antibacterial properties. It relieves many types of skin irritations.
- Spray or dab pure aloe vera juice (chilled feels especially nice) directly on bites. It soothes the skin and relieves itchiness.

Lemony Bugs-Away Spray

This light-textured repellent leaves your skin feeling fresh and clean and scented with a lingering, lemony aroma enjoyed by all.

2 cups witch hazel
1 teaspoon vegetable glycerin
20 drops citronella essential oil
20 drops lemongrass essential oil

RECOMMENDED FOR: *all skin types except very sensitive*
USE: *as needed*
PREP TIME: *approximately 5 to 10 minutes*
BLENDING TOOLS: *shake bottle before each use*
STORE IN: *plastic or glass spritzer bottle*
YIELD: *approximately 2 cups*

Combine all ingredients in a 16-ounce glass or plastic spray bottle or two 8-ounce spray bottles. Shake the mixture vigorously to blend. The essential oils will tend to separate out and sit on top (like oil in salad dressing), but this does not affect the product.

No refrigeration is required, but for maximum potency and freshness, please store the blend away from light and heat. Use within 1 year.

APPLICATION TIPS: Shake well immediately before use. Apply liberally to skin as needed — approximately every 15 to 20 minutes. Use common sense in application: Don't spray directly into your eyes, nose, or mouth.

Note: This mix may stain white or pale-colored clothing.

Herbal Insect-Deterrent Potpourri for a Fragrant, Bug-Free Home

Unless you have damaging infestations of fleas, termites, carpenter ants, or other destructive insects in and around your home, try an old-fashioned way of ridding your living quarters of nasty pesky moths, mosquitoes, ants, spiders, silverfish, earwigs, and flies: Various pungent herbs have been used for centuries to chase away existing bugs as well as to prevent bugs and flying insects from entering homes and storage spaces and setting up shop. They're inexpensive, effective, non-toxic, and wonderfully pleasing to the senses.

Simply fill small bowls or muslin bags with dried rosemary, thyme, lavender buds, cedar chips, lemongrass, peppermint, and tansy (or any combination you desire) and place the herbs in food pantries, under beds and bathroom sinks, in clothing closets and drawers, on the kitchen counter, near open windows, and close to heating and cooling vents. Add a drop or two of essential oil of cedar, peppermint, rosemary, citronella, or lemongrass to your potpourri bowl or bag to enhance its bug repelling properties.

And remember the six things that bugs love best: moisture or standing water, warmth, exposed food, sticky countertops and floors, rotten wood, and the aroma of sweat and human exhalation. Strive to keep your home in good repair and as clean and dry as possible so it won't be inviting to pests.

Resources

Mail-Order Suppliers for Raw Materials, Packaging, and Natural Personal Care Products

Aphrodisia Herb Shoppe
212-989-6440
www.aphrodisiaherbshoppe.com
Extensive line of herbal products, including essential oils, herbs, spices, natural soaps, bath salts, base oils, and cosmetic clays. If you're in New York City, plan to visit this herbal emporium.

Aroma Therapeutix
800-308-6284
www.aromatherapeutix.com
Offers single essential oils and oil blends, some packaging, soaps, herbal body and health care products, small muslin bags, and more.

Aroma Vera
800-669-9514
www.aromavera.com
Supplier of essential oils; base oils; and natural skin, hair, and body care products.

Aubrey Organics
800-282-7394
www.aubrey-organics.com
Manufacturer of chemical-free, natural skin, hair, and body care products, cosmetics, and fragrances.

Aura Cacia
800-437-3301
www.auracacia.com
Supplier of essential oils, base oils, and natural skin and body care products. Part of Frontier Natural Products Co-op.

Avena Botanicals
866-282-8362
www.avenabotanicals.com
Retailer of organic tinctures; elixirs; glycerites; herbal teas; herbs; essential oils; chemical-free, natural skin and body care; children's herbal health care; herbal pet care products; and books.

The Baker's Catalogue, King
Arthur Flour
800-827-6836
www.bakerscatalogue.com
Fabulous flavorings, specialty bake-
ware, measuring tools, seasonings,
tasty flours, ingredient scales, and
more.

Banyan Botanicals
800-953-6424
www.banyanbotanicals.com
Offers traditional, hard-to-find
Ayurvedic herbs, base oils, and body
care and health products.

Bindi
800-952-4634
www.bindi.com
Supplier of natural and chemical-free
Ayurvedic skin, hair, body, and oral
care products.

Cape Bottle Co., Inc.
888-833-6307 or 508-833-6307
www.netbottle.com
Offers a wide variety of glass, plastic,
and tin packaging.

Champlain Valley Apiaries
800-841-7334
www.champlainvalleyhoney.com
Fresh beeswax, beeswax candles, raw
honey, maple syrup, and a few bees-
wax- or honey-based natural body
care products.

Dr. Hauschka Skin Care, Inc.
800-247-9907
www.drhauschka.com
Organic, holistic, chemical-free skin,
hair, and body care products and
cosmetics. Ingredients are biodynamically grown, and products are
homeopathically prepared.

Ecco Bella
877-696-2220
www.eccobella.com
Organic, natural, and chemical-free
skin, hair, and body care products,
cosmetics, and fragrances.

The Essential Oil Company
503-872-8772
www.essentialoil.com
Pure aromatherapy essential oils,
massage oils, fragrance oils, soapmak-
ing supplies, and unscented incense.

Frontier Natural Products Co-op
800-669-3275
www.frontiercoop.com
A personal care crafter's paradise!
Maintains a large inventory of essential oils; base oils; natural and organic herbs; spices; teas; dried foods and mixes; cosmetic clays; beeswax; and natural skin, hair, and body care products.

Honey Gardens Apiaries, Inc.
888-303-4429
www.honeygardens.com
Supplier of fresh beeswax, beeswax candles, raw honey, a few handmade herbal skin care products, and delicious honey-herbal blend health-promoting syrups.

Jean's Greens
888-845-8327
www.jeansgreens.com
A range of wonderful herb products, teas, herbs, essential oils, packaging supplies, beeswax, base oils, butters, clays, books, and more.

The Jojoba Company
800-256-5622 or 207-832-4401
www.jojobacompany.com
Certified organic, unrefined, superior-quality jojoba oil. Pricing information available.

Lavender Lane Forever
888-593-4400
www.lavenderlane.com
Supplies essential, base, and fragrance oils; waxes; butters; cosmetic clays; books; and a wide array of packaging supplies.

Lavera
877-528-3727
www.lavera-usa.com
Organic, natural, and chemical-free skin, hair, body, and oral care products and cosmetics.

Liberty Natural Products
800-289-8427
www.libertynatural.com
Supplier of just about every botanical ingredient you can imagine. A personal care crafter's dream! Also offers packaging supplies, flavorings, soap supplies, and more.

LorAnn Oils, Inc.
888-456-7266
www.lorannoils.com
Fine flavorings, essential oils, some packaging supplies, body care crafting kits and supplies, and base oils.

Mountain Rose Herbs
800-879-3337
www.mountainroseherbs.com
Carries everything you could possibly want related to herbs: seeds; books; essential and base oils; raw ingredients; packaging; herbal health aids; and natural skin, hair, and body care products.

MyChelle Dermaceuticals, LLC
800-447-2076
www.mychelleusa.com
Nontoxic, therapeutic skin and body care products.

Original Swiss Aromatics
415-479-9120
www.originalswissaromatics.com
Superior quality, therapeutic-grade, authentic essential oils derived from ethically wild-crafted or organically grown plants. Also supplies facial oils and massage and body oils.

Simplers Botanical Company
800-652-7646
www.simplers.com
Genuine and authentic therapeutic-grade essential oils ethically wild-crafted or organically or biodynamically grown. Superior quality. Also carries natural first-aid oils, hydrosols, perfume oils, infused herbal oils, and herbal extracts.

Stephanie Tourles
www.herbalsoapandskincare.com
Author, licensed holistic esthetician, herbalist, aromatherapist.

Weleda, Inc.
800-241-1030
www.usa.weleda.com
Organic, natural, and chemical-free skin, hair, body, and oral care products. Homeopathic medicines.

Zack Woods Herb Farm
802-888-7278
www.zackwoodsherbs.com
Offers 35 species of organically grown fresh and dried herbs.

Herb and Garden Seeds and Gardening Supplies

The Cook's Garden
800-457-9703
www.cooksgarden.com
Untreated and often organic vegetable, flower, and herb seeds; plants; books; gardening supplies; and a few unique bottles, jars, and tins.

Pinetree Garden Seeds
207-926-3400
www.superseeds.com
Offers flower, vegetable, and herb seeds; plants; gardening supplies; books; body care kits; and some natural skin care products.

Seeds of Change
888-762-7333
www.seedsofchange.com
Offers 100 percent–certified organic, GMO-free, open-pollinated vegetable, flower, and herb seeds; gardening supplies; greenhouses; some seedlings; books; and posters. It offers many heirloom, rare, and traditional seed varieties as well.

Territorial Seed Company
800-626-0866
www.territorial-seed.com
Offers flower, vegetable, and herb seeds; plants; gardening supplies; and books.

Herb Associations and Correspondence Courses

American Herb Association
530-265-9552
www.ahaherb.com
Available through this organization is a comprehensive listing of herb schools, seminars, programs, correspondence courses, and herb suppliers throughout the United States. I urge you to obtain a copy. They also offer a fabulous quarterly newsletter that I highly recommend to any herb enthusiast.

Australasian College of Health Sciences
800-487-8839
www.achs.edu
Specializes in accredited, online, holistic health education.

Clayton College of Natural Health
800-995-4590
www.ccnh.edu
Offers various natural health and
herbal correspondence courses.

Dominion Herbal College
888-342-1926 or 604-433-1926
www.dominionherbal.com
Offers herbal correspondence
courses.

East West School of Herbology
800-717-5010
www.planetherbs.com
Offers books and herbal correspondence courses based on traditional
Chinese herbal medicine and Orien-
tal healing systems.

International Aromatherapy and
Herb Association
602-938-4439
www.aromaherbshow.com
Publisher of *Making Scents* magazine,
which covers in-depth topics on
essential oils, herbs, healing foods,
and healthy living. Highly recommended. A good educational resource
for the personal care crafter. Some
free articles from back issues are
available.

Pacific Institute of Aromatherapy
415-479-9120
www.pacificinstituteofaromatherapy.com
Offers an in-depth correspondence
course on aromatherapy.

The School of Natural Healing
800-372-8255
www.snh.cc
Offers comprehensive herbal correspondence courses based on Western
herbalism.

The Science and Art of Herbalism
with Rosemary Gladstar
802-479-9825
www.sagemountain.com
Contact for course information.
Rosemary offers a lovely, in-depth,
beautifully written correspondence
course for the beginner or
intermediate-level Western herbalist.

Suggested Reading

This list includes resources for this book, as well as selections from my personal library.

Alt, Carol. *Eating in the Raw: A Beginner's Guide to Getting Slimmer, Feeling Healthier, and Looking Younger the Raw-Food Way.* New York: Clarkson Potter, 2004.

Balch, Phyllis A., and James F. Balch. *Prescription for Nutritional Healing,* third edition. New York: Avery, 2000.

Cousin, Pierre Jean. *Facelift at Your Fingertips: An Aromatherapy Massage Program for Healthy Skin and a Younger Face.* North Adams, Mass.: Storey Publishing, 2000.

Duke, James A. *The Green Pharmacy: Anti-Aging Prescriptions.* Emmaus, Pa.: Rodale, 2001.

Fairley, Josephine, and Sarah Stacey. *Feel Fabulous Forever: The Anti-Aging Health and Beauty Bible.* Woodstock, N.Y.: Overlook Press, 1999.

Falconi, Dina. *Earthly Bodies and Heavenly Hair: Natural and Healthy Personal Care for Every Body.* Woodstock, N.Y.: Ceres Press, 1998.

Furjanic, Sheila, and Jacqueline Flynn, editors. *Milady's Art and Science of Nail Technology,* revised edition. Albany, N.Y.: Milady Publishing, 1992.

Gerson, Joel. *Milady's Standard Textbook for Professional Estheticians,* eighth edition. Albany, N.Y.: Thomson Learning, 1999.

Gladstar, Rosemary. *Herbal Healing for Women.* New York: Simon and Schuster, 1993.

———. *Herbs for Longevity and Well-Being.* North Adams, Mass.: Storey Books, 1999.

———. *Rosemary Gladstar's Family Herbal: A Guide to Living Life with Energy, Health, and Vitality.* North Adams, Mass.: Storey Publishing, 2001.

Haddon, Dayle. *Ageless Beauty.* New York: Hyperion, 1998.

Hampton, Aubrey, and Susan Hussey. *The Take Charge Beauty Book: The Natural Guide to Beautiful Hair and Skin.* Tampa, Fla.: Organica Press, 2000.

Hofstein, Riquette. *Grow Hair in 12 Weeks.* New York: Crown, 1988.

James, Kat. *The Truth about Beauty: Transform Your Looks and Your Life from the Inside Out.* Hillsboro, Oreg.: Beyond Words Publishing, 2003.

Janssen, Mary Beth. *Naturally Healthy Hair: Herbal Treatments and Daily Care for Fabulous Hair.* North Adams, Mass.: Storey Publishing, 1999.

Keville, Kathi. *Herbs for Health and Healing: A Drug-Free Guide to Prevention and Cure.* Emmaus, Pa.: Rodale, 1996.

Kloss, Jethro. *Back to Eden.* Santa Barbara, Calif.: Woodbridge Press, 1939.

Knowles, Elizabeth, editor. *The Oxford Dictionary of Quotations,* fifth edition. New York: Oxford University Press, 1999.

Long, Jim. *Herbal Cosmetics.* Oak Grove, Ark.: Long Creek Herbs, 1996.

———. *Just for Men.* Oak Grove, Ark.: Long Creek Herbs, 1992.

Lust, John B. *The Herb Book.* New York: Bantam Books, 1974.

Maria, Donna. *Making Aromatherapy Creams and Lotions: 101 Natural Formulas to Revitalize and Nourish Your Skin.* North Adams, Mass.: Storey Publishing, 2000.

Massey, Lorraine, with Deborah Chiel. *Curly Girl: More than Just Hair . . . It's an Attitude.* New York: Workman, 2001.

McCarter, Robert, and Elizabeth McCarter. *Nutrition and the Skin, The Life Science Health System, Part 12, Natural Hygiene: A Better Way of Living, Lesson 61.* Austin, Tex.: College of Life Science, 1983.

Ody, Penelope. *The Complete Medicinal Herbal.* New York: Dorling Kindersley, 1993.

Phillips, Nancy, and Michael Phillips. *The Village Herbalist: Sharing Plant Medicines with Family and Community.* White River Junction, Vt.: Chelsea Green, 2001.

Pugliese, Peter T. *Physiology of the Skin.* Carol Stream, Ill.: Allured Publishing, 1996.

Sarfati, Lydia. *Repêchage Professional Skin Care Manual.* New York: Sarkli-Repêchage, 1984.

Schneider, Anny. *Wild Medicinal Plants.* Mechanicsburg, Pa.: Stackpole Books, 2002.

Soltanoff, Jack. *Natural Healing.* New York: Warner Books, 1988.

Soule, Deb. *A Woman's Book of Herbs.* New York: Carol, 1998.

Stephan-Wise, Ouidad. *Curl Talk.* New York: Three Rivers Press, 2002.

Tisserand, Maggie. *Essence of Love: Fragrance, Aphrodisiacs, and Aromatherapy for Lovers.* New York: HarperCollins, 1993.

Tourles, Stephanie. *50 Simple Ways to Pamper Yourself.* North Adams, Mass.: Storey Publishing, 1999.

Weed, Susun S. *Breast Cancer? Breast Health!: The Wise Woman Way.* Woodstock, N.Y.: Ash Tree Publishing, 1996.

Weinberg, Norma Pasekoff. *Natural Hand Care: Herbal Treatments and Simple Techniques for Healthy Hands and Nails.* North Adams, Mass.: Storey Publishing, 1998.

Worwood, Valerie Ann. *The Complete Book of Essential Oils and Aromatherapy.* San Rafael, Calif.: New World Library, 1991.

———. *How to Feel Fabulous Today!: 250 Simple and Natural Ways to Achieve Spiritual, Emotional, and Physical Well-Being.* North Adams, Mass.: Storey Publishing, 2001.

———. *Natural Foot Care: Herbal Treatments, Massage, and Exercises for Healthy Feet.* North Adams, Mass.: Storey Publishing, 1998.

———. *Naturally Healthy Skin: Tips and Techniques for a Lifetime of Radiant Skin.* North Adams, Mass.: Storey Publishing, 1999.

Index

Other Storey Titles You Will Enjoy

50 Simple Ways to Pamper Yourself, by Stephanie Tourles.
Easy, inspiring ideas and simple recipes for facials, massages,
baths, soaks, and other techniques for relieving everyday stress.
144 pages. Paper. ISBN-13: 978-1-58017-201-3.

365 Ways to Energize Mind, Body & Soul, by Stephanie Tourles.
An fun idea-a-day book that's filled with natural ways to stay
alert and upbeat.
384 pages. Paper. ISBN-13: 978-1-58017-331-5.

The Aromatherapy Companion, by Victoria H. Edwards.
The most comprehensive aromatherapy guide, filled with profiles
of essential oils and recipes for beauty, health, and well-being.
288 pages. Paper. ISBN-13: 978-1-58017-150-2.

Natural Foot Care, by Stephanie Tourles.
A comprehensive handbook of natural, homemade herbal
treatments, massage techniques, and exercises for healthy feet.
192 pages. Paper. ISBN-13: 978-1-58017-054-3.

Naturally Healthy Skin, by Stephanie Tourles.
A total reference about caring for all types of skin, with recipes,
techniques, and practical advice.
208 pages. Paper. ISBN-13: 978-1-58017-130-4.

These and other books from Storey Publishing are available
wherever quality books are sold or by calling 1-800-441-5700.
Visit us at *www.storey.com.*